PROLOG

Female Pelvic Medicine and Reconstructive Surgery

Critique Book

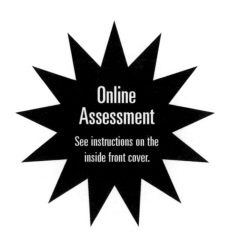

Online Assessment

See instructions on the inside front cover.

The American College of
Obstetricians and Gynecologists
WOMEN'S HEALTH CARE PHYSICIANS

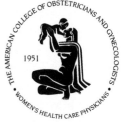

ISBN 978-1-934984-55-0

45/0

The American College of Obstetricians and Gynecologists
409 12th Street, SW
PO Box 96920
Washington, DC 20090-6920

Contributors

PROLOG Editorial and Advisory Committee

CHAIR

Ronald T. Burkman Jr, MD
  Professor of Obstetrics and
    Gynecology
  Department of Obstetrics and
    Gynecology
  Tufts University School of Medicine
  Baystate Medical Center
  Springfield, Massachusetts

MEMBERS

Louis Weinstein, MD
  Past Paul A. and Eloise B. Bowers
    Professor and Chair
  Department of Obstetrics and
    Gynecology
  Thomas Jefferson University
  Philadelphia, Pennsylvania

PROLOG Task Force for *Female Pelvic Medicine and Reconstructive Surgery*

CHAIR

Kimberly Kenton MD, MS
  Chief and Fellowship Program Director
  Division of Female Pelvic Medicine &
    Reconstructive Surgery
  Departments of Obstetrics & Gynecology
    and Urology
  Northwestern University Feinberg School
    of Medicine
  Chicago, Illinois

MEMBERS

Melinda G. Abernethy, MD, MPH
  Assistant Professor
  Division of Female Pelvic Medicine and
    Gynecologic Surgery
  Department of Gynecology and
    Obstetrics
  Johns Hopkins Hospital
  Baltimore, Maryland

Jennifer Anger, MD, MPH
  Associate Professor of Urology
  Associate Director of Urological
    Research
  Urologic Reconstruction, Urodynamics,
    and Female Urology
  Cedars-Sinai Medical Center
  Beverly Hills, California

Cara Grimes, MD, MAS
  Assistant Professor of Obstetrics and
    Gynecology
  Female Pelvic Medicine and
    Reconstructive Surgery
  Gynecologic Specialty Surgery
  Columbia University Medical Center
  New York, New York

Catherine Matthews, MD
  Professor
  Department of Obstetrics & Gynecology
    and Urology
  Wake Forest Baptist Health
  Winston Salem, North Carolina

Continued on next page

CONFLICT OF INTEREST DISCLOSURE

This PROLOG unit was developed under the direction of the PROLOG Advisory Committee and the Task Force for *Female Pelvic Medicine and Reconstructive Surgery*. PROLOG is planned and produced in accordance with the Standards for Enduring Materials of the Accreditation Council for Continuing Medical Education. Any discussion of unapproved use of products is clearly cited in the appropriate critique.

Current guidelines state that continuing medical education (CME) providers must ensure that CME activities are free from the control of any commercial interest. The task force and advisory committee members declare that neither they nor any business associate nor any member of their immediate families has material interest, financial interest, or other relationships with any company manufacturing commercial products relative to the topics included in this publication or with any provider of commercial services discussed in the unit. All potential conflicts have been resolved through the American College of Obstetricians and Gynecologists' mechanism for resolving potential and real conflicts of interest.

Preface

Purpose

PROLOG (Personal Review of Learning in Obstetrics and Gynecology) is a voluntary, strictly confidential self-evaluation program. PROLOG was developed specifically as a personal study resource for the practicing obstetrician–gynecologist. It is presented as a self-assessment mechanism that, with its accompanying performance information, should assist the physician in designing a personal, self-directed lifelong learning program. It may be used as a valuable study tool, a reference guide, and a means of attaining up-to-date information in the specialty. The content is carefully selected and presented in multiple-choice questions that are clinically oriented. The questions are designed to stimulate and challenge physicians in areas of medical care that they confront in their practices or when they work as consultant obstetrician–gynecologists.

PROLOG also provides the American College of Obstetricians and Gynecologists (the College) with one mechanism to identify the educational needs of the Fellows. Individual scores are reported only to the participant; however, cumulative performance data and evaluation comments obtained for each PROLOG unit help determine the direction for future educational programs offered by the College.

Process

The PROLOG series offers the most current information available in five areas of the specialty: obstetrics, gynecology and surgery, reproductive endocrinology and infertility, gynecologic oncology and critical care, and patient management in the office. A new PROLOG unit is produced annually, addressing one of those subject areas. The College also produces volumes of PROLOG that concentrate on additional specialty areas, such as *Female Pelvic Medicine and Reconstructive Surgery*.

Each unit of PROLOG represents the efforts of a task force of subject experts under the supervision of an advisory committee. PROLOG sets forth current information as viewed by recognized authorities in the field of women's health. This educational resource does not define a standard of care, nor is it intended to dictate an exclusive course of management. It presents recognized methods and techniques of clinical practice for consideration by obstetrician–gynecologists to incorporate in their practices. Variations of practice that take into account the needs of the individual patient, resources, and the limitations that are special to the institution or type of practice may be appropriate.

Each unit of PROLOG is presented as a two-part set, with performance information and cognate credit available to those who choose to submit their answers electronically for confidential scoring. Participants can work through the unit at their own pace, choosing to use PROLOG as a closed or open assessment. The Critique Book provides the rationale for correct and incorrect options, and current, accessible references.

Continuing Medical Education Credit

ACCME Accreditation
The American College of Obstetricians and Gynecologists is accredited by the Accreditation Council for Continuing Medical Education (ACCME) to provide continuing medical education for physicians.

AMA PRA Category 1 Credit(s)™
The American College of Obstetricians and Gynecologists designates this enduring material for a maximum of 14 *AMA PRA Category 1 Credits*™. Physicians should claim only the credit commensurate with the extent of their participation in the activity.

College Cognate Credit(s)

The American College of Obstetricians and Gynecologists designates this enduring material for a maximum of 14 Category 1 College Cognate Credits. The College has a reciprocity agreement with the American Medical Association that allows *AMA PRA Category 1 Credits*™ to be equivalent to College Cognate Credits.

Participants who submit their assessment and achieve a passing score will be credited with 14 hours and will receive a Performance Report that provides a comparison of their scores with the scores of a sample group of physicians who have taken the unit as an examination. An individual may request credit only once for each unit.

Credit for PROLOG *Female Pelvic Medicine and Reconstructive Surgery* is initially available through December 2018. During that year, the unit will be reevaluated. If the content remains current, credit is extended for an additional 3 years, with credit for the unit automatically withdrawn after December 2021.

New: Electronic Assessment for CME Credit

For this unit, the CME Assessment can only be submitted electronically. Assessment results must be above 80% to achieve a passing score and attain CME credit. To access the online assessment, please visit www.acog.org/PROLOGexam. Test results and the CME certificate will be available upon completion of the examination.

If you purchased a print book, use the key code located on the inside front cover of the Critique Book and follow the directions provided. If you purchased an eBook, please follow the instructions online to purchase and access the assessment.

Conclusion

PROLOG was developed specifically as a personal study resource for the practicing obstetrician–gynecologist. It is presented as a self-assessment mechanism that, with its accompanying performance information, should assist the physician in designing a personal, self-directed learning program. The many quality resources developed by the College, as detailed each year in the College's *Publications and Educational Materials Catalog*, are available to help fulfill the educational interests and needs that have been identified. PROLOG is not intended as a substitute for the certification or recertification programs of the American Board of Obstetrics and Gynecology.

PROLOG CME SCHEDULE	
Gynecologic Oncology and Critical Care, Sixth Edition	Credit through 2016
Patient Management in the Office, Sixth Edition	Reevaluated in 2014– Credit through 2017
Obstetrics, Seventh Edition	Reevaluated in 2015– Credit through 2018
Gynecology and Surgery, Seventh Edition	Reevaluated in 2016– Credit through 2019
Reproductive Endocrinology and Infertility, Seventh Edition	Reevaluated in 2017– Credit through 2020
Gynecologic Oncology and Critical Care, Seventh Edition	Reevaluated in 2018– Credit through 2021
Female Pelvic Medicine and Reconstructive Surgery	Reevaluated in 2018– Credit through 2021

PROLOG Objectives

PROLOG is a voluntary, strictly confidential, personal continuing education resource that is designed to be stimulating and enjoyable. By participating in PROLOG, obstetrician–gynecologists will be able to do the following:

- Review and update clinical knowledge.
- Recognize areas of knowledge and practice in which they excel, be stimulated to explore other areas of the specialty, and identify areas requiring further study.
- Plan continuing education activities in light of identified strengths and deficiencies.
- Compare and relate present knowledge and skills with those of other participants.
- Obtain continuing medical education credit, if desired.
- Have complete personal control of the setting and of the pace of the experience.

The obstetrician–gynecologist who completes *Female Pelvic Medicine and Reconstructive Surgery* will be able to

- discuss normal pelvic anatomy and physiology and how alterations in anatomy and physiology contribute to development of pelvic floor disorders.
- identify the pathophysiologic and epidemiologic factors that contribute to pelvic floor disorders in women.
- associate symptom bother and quality of life effect of different pelvic floor disorders, determine appropriate diagnostic workups, and select accurate diagnoses.
- associate pelvic floor symptoms with corresponding signs on examination and testing to ensure accurate diagnoses.
- discuss the alternative surgical and nonsurgical treatment options for pelvic floor disorders and identify common complications of therapy.
- apply knowledge of anatomy and appropriate surgical techniques in the surgical treatment of pelvic floor disorders.

Female Pelvic Medicine and Reconstructive Surgery includes the following topics (item numbers appear in parentheses):

SCREENING AND DIAGNOSIS
Nerve entrapment with uterosacral ligament suspension (47)
Office evaluation of incontinence (8)
Pelvic anatomy (1)
Rectal prolapse (41)
Spinal cord lesion (34)
Stress urinary incontinence (13)
Vaginal agenesis (33)
Vertebral discitis (46)

MEDICAL MANAGEMENT
Aging and hormonal effects on the pelvic floor (6)
Bowel complications after robotic sacrocolpopexy (30)
Cystoscopy (44)
Detrusor sphincter dyssynergia (43)
Fecal incontinence (37)
Mesh complications (22, 27)
Midurethral slings (50)
Neuromodulation for urgency urinary incontinence (16)
Nocturia (40)
Occult stress incontinence in patient with prolapse (23)
Painful bladder syndrome (24)

A complete subject matter index appears at the end of the Critique Book.

1

Pelvic anatomy

A 17-year-old girl comes to your office for evaluation of a vaginal wall cyst that had been noted by her primary care provider. She is asymptomatic and has no comorbidities. She is not sexually active and reports regular menses. She experienced menarche at age 12 years. Pelvic examination reveals a painless, fluctuant, fluid-filled 6-cm mass on the left lateral vagina, approximately 4 cm cephalad to the hymenal ring (Fig. 1-1). The most likely diagnosis is

        (A) urethral diverticulum
*   (B) mesonephric duct remnant
        (C) Bartholin cyst
        (D) pronephric duct remnant
        (E) Skene gland cyst

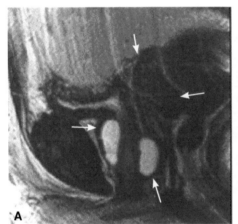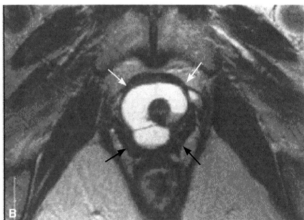

FIG. 1-1. Urethral diverticulum as seen on magnetic resonance imaging. (Reprinted with permission of Anderson Publishing Ltd. from Hubert J, Bergin D. Imaging the female pelvis: when should MRI be considered? Appl Radiol 2008;37:9–24. Copyright Anderson Publishing, Ltd.)

This patient's cyst is consistent with a Gartner duct cyst, which is the embryonic remnant of the mesonephric or wolffian duct. Gartner duct cysts commonly are found along the posterior or lateral vagina and are filled with serous or mucinous fluid. Some females have Gartner duct cysts in adolescence and are unable to insert a tampon or experience pain with tampon insertion; however, many women are asymptomatic. Management can be expectant or include excision or marsupialization, based on the patient's symptoms.

Urethral diverticula are cystic structures typically seen within the distal 3 cm of the anterior vaginal wall, arising from the posterior urethra. They are seen most commonly in adult women and are rare in children and adolescents. Although they can be asymptomatic, many urethral diverticula occur along with urinary incontinence or postvoid dribbling, dysuria, or dyspareunia. Magnetic resonance imaging is the criterion standard to confirm the diagnosis of a urethral diverticulum.

Bartholin gland ducts secrete mucus and serve to lubricate the vaginal introitus. The ducts empty into the vaginal vestibule at the 4 o'clock and 8 o'clock positions distal to the hymenal ring. The location of the mass in this patient is not consistent with a Bartholin cyst.

The pronephros is the first, nonfunctional progenitor of the kidney that appears and regresses in the fourth week of embryonic development. Without regression of the pronephric duct, normal kidney development cannot continue.

Skene glands are periurethral glands that are responsible for lubrication and are the closest female analog to the male prostate gland. Skene ducts can become

* Indicates correct answer.
Note: See Appendix A for a table of normal values for laboratory tests.

1

obstructed, leading to Skene gland swelling and pain. The diagnosis of Skene gland cyst can be confirmed by physical examination, given that the glands are located within the anterior vaginal wall lateral to the urethral meatus.

Baggish MS, Karram MM. Atlas of pelvic anatomy and gynecologic surgery. 3rd ed. Philadelphia (PA): Elsevier Saunders; 2011.

Foley CL, Greenwell TJ, Gardiner RA. Urethral diverticula in females. BJU Int 2011;108:20–3.

Sadler TW. Urogenital system. In: Langman's medical embryology. 13th ed. Philadelphia (PA): Wolters Kluwer Health; 2015. p. 250–77.

Wai CY, Corton MM, Miller M, Sailors J, Schaffer JI. Multiple vaginal wall cysts: diagnosis and surgical management. Obstet Gynecol 2004;103:1099–102.

2

Pelvic organ prolapse repair

A 65-year-old woman, gravida 3, para 3, has stage III anterior vaginal wall prolapse. The surgical repair that is most likely to resolve her underlying pelvic support defect is

      (A) anterior repair with midline plication
      (B) anterior repair with insertion of polypropylene mesh
      (C) bilateral paravaginal repair
*   (D) anterior repair with sacrospinous ligament fixation

Approximately 13% of women will undergo pelvic organ prolapse repair by age 80 years. Pelvic organ prolapse is multifactorial in etiology. The most common risk factors are vaginal childbirth, aging, and higher body mass index. The typical symptom of pelvic organ prolapse is a vaginal bulge. Many women do not report the bulge as bothersome until it protrudes beyond the hymen.

The principal support mechanisms of the pelvic floor include the levator ani muscle complex (puborectalis, pubococcygeus, and iliococcygeus) and the connective tissue attachments of the pelvic organs, commonly referred to as endopelvic fascia. The levator ani are tonically contracted muscles that reduce the size of the genital hiatus and provide a stable platform on which the viscera rest. Levator ani injury, in the form of avulsion or denervation, results in the widening and ballooning down of the pelvic floor. Three-dimensional ultrasonography and magnetic resonance imaging have demonstrated a strong correlation between large levator ani defects, increased size of the genital hiatus, and advanced prolapse.

The ligamentous support to the vagina is classically described as three levels of support:

- Level I—Support at the vaginal apex where the cardinal–uterosacral ligament complex is attached to the pubocervical and rectovaginal fascial rings and suspends the apex of the vagina
- Level II—Midvaginal lateral support where the pubocervical fascia is attached laterally to the arcus tendineus fasciae pelvis

- Level III—Support via the distal vaginal attachments to the perineal membrane ventrally and perineal body dorsally

Because gynecologic surgeons are not equipped to surgically address levator ani muscle defects, the intraoperative focus traditionally has been on repairing the endopelvic fascial defects and attachments. However, it is necessary to address all levels of compromised pelvic support to facilitate surgical success.

In randomized trials, poor success rates of 40–60% have been reported for isolated anterior colporrhaphy, in which the anterior fibromuscular wall of the vagina is plicated in the midline over a central defect. Studies using magnetic resonance imaging have demonstrated the critical interplay between anterior and apical pelvic support: 65% of women who present with anterior wall prolapse have loss of level I (apical) support. Because this loss of support is not addressed at the time of surgery, it likely has contributed to such high rates of surgical failure with traditional anterior repair. The described patient is unlikely to have an isolated central anterior prolapse and, therefore, isolated anterior repair, with or without the use of mesh, is unlikely to address her comprehensive pelvic floor defect.

Paravaginal defect repairs involve reattaching the pubocervical fascia to the arcus tendineus fasciae pelvis and, overall, have a higher success rate than isolated central plication. Although this technique does provide some support to the vaginal apex, particularly if the deepest stitch is placed just above the ischial spine, it will not address a central anterior wall defect. Paravaginal repair also has been associated with higher rates of surgical complications than midline plication.

Polypropylene mesh in the anterior compartment has been associated with improved objective outcomes, but not subjective outcomes, compared with standard anterior colporrhaphy. Whether the mesh insert is designed to address a concomitant apical defect, however, has a significant effect on overall surgical success. Mesh kits for the anterior compartment that attach to the sacrospinous ligaments are able to address the high rate of concomitant defects that exist in the anterior and apical compartments. To date, no long-term studies have been reported of mesh kits designed to address anterior and apical defects. A mesh product that is merely an overlay to a central repair will not be sufficient to address a concomitant apical defect.

The sacrospinous ligaments, uterosacral ligaments, and iliococcygeus fascia are the three options that can be employed vaginally for apical support. The advantages of the sacrospinous and iliococcygeus options are that they are extraperitoneal and do not carry the risks of ureteric injury. The uterosacral ligaments offer the most anatomic support of the vagina. In a recent randomized trial comparing uterosacral with sacrospinous fixation, there was no difference in overall success or complication rates. In cases of a large anterior wall defect, reduction of the vaginal apex alone may not be sufficient to provide normal support, and typically, a central plication is required in addition to either a uterosacral or a sacrospinous ligament fixation to complete the procedure.

Barber MD, Brubaker L, Burgio KL, Richter HE, Nygaard I, Weidner AC, et al. Comparison of 2 transvaginal surgical approaches and perioperative behavioral therapy for apical vaginal prolapse: the OPTIMAL randomized trial. Eunice Kennedy Shriver National Institute of Child Health and Human Development Pelvic Floor Disorders Network [published erratum appears in JAMA 2015;313:2287]. JAMA 2014;311:1023–34.

Lowder JL, Park AJ, Ellison R, Ghetti C, Moalli P, Zyczynski H, et al. The role of apical vaginal support in the appearance of anterior and posterior vaginal prolapse. Obstet Gynecol 2008;111:152–7.

Maher C, Feiner B, Baessler K, Schmid C. Surgical management of pelvic organ prolapse in women. Cochrane Database of Systematic Reviews 2013, Issue 4. Art. No.: CD004014. DOI: 10.1002/14651858. CD004014.pub5.

3

Mode of delivery and pelvic floor dysfunction

A 30-year-old woman, gravida 1, para 0, at 28 weeks of gestation, asks for your advice in regard to mode of delivery. She is contemplating a cesarean delivery by maternal request because she is concerned about pelvic floor dysfunction. You advise her that the immediate postpartum risk that cesarean delivery may help to reduce is

* (A) urinary incontinence
   (B) anal incontinence
   (C) pelvic organ prolapse
   (D) levator spasms

Cesarean delivery by maternal request is primary, prelabor cesarean delivery at the request of the pregnant woman in the absence of any maternal or fetal indications. It is considered to be a subset of elective cesarean delivery, which refers to planned cesarean delivery for certain maternal or fetal indications. From 2003 to 2009, the rate of primary cesarean delivery in the United States increased from 14.4% to 21.7%, with cesarean delivery by maternal request accounting for approximately 8% of the total increase. Most patients (64% in one study) who request an elective cesarean delivery refer to tocophobia or fear of labor as the basis for their request. Other reasons include concerns about the health of the fetus, the patient's own life, or both (28%); heredity for complicated birth among female relatives (20%); fear of pain during a vaginal delivery (18%); history of sexual violence (11%); depression (11%); and anxiety regarding emergency cesarean delivery (10%).

Pregnancy itself appears to be a risk factor for urinary incontinence, and it is unclear how much this risk is mediated by mode of delivery. In a cohort study of 523 women monitored for 12 months postpartum, vaginal delivery was noted to be an independent risk factor for the development of urinary incontinence (odds ratio [OR], 2.18; $P=.006$). The Epidemiology of Incontinence study, a large population-based study of 27,900 Norwegian women, also found a higher risk (2.2-fold) for urinary incontinence among premenopausal women who delivered vaginally compared with premenopausal women who delivered by cesarean delivery. However, the possible protective effect of cesarean delivery was not found among older women (aged 65–74 years).

To date, no randomized controlled trial has addressed the use of cesarean delivery to decrease the postpartum risk of pelvic floor disorders. The Term Breech Trial assigned 1,159 women with term breech fetuses to either a planned cesarean or planned vaginal delivery and measured rates of postpartum urinary incontinence. The investigators found a decreased relative risk (RR) for urinary incontinence among the planned cesarean delivery group at 3 months postpartum (RR, 0.62; 95% confidence interval [CI], 0.41–0.93) based on a self-reported history of incontinence symptoms over the past 7 days. However, this significance did not persist at 2 years (RR, 0.81; 95% CI, 0.61–1.1). Furthermore, higher rates of incontinence were noted at 2 years compared with the rates at 3 months for planned cesarean delivery and planned vaginal delivery (17.8% and 21.8% at 2 years versus 4.5% and 7.3% at 3 months, respectively). The higher rates may be due to differences in data collection because the 2-year respondents were asked to report symptoms over the past 3–6 months.

A nested case–control study based on the Swedish Hospital Discharge Registry found a protective association between cesarean delivery and admission for pelvic organ prolapse surgery (OR, 0.18; 95% CI, 0.16–0.20). A longitudinal cohort study of 1,011 women in the United States found a significantly greater chance of prolapse to or beyond the hymen among women who had vaginal deliveries versus those who had cesarean deliveries (OR, 5.6; 95% CI, 2.2–14.7). However, these women were enrolled 5–10 years after the birth of their first child. No data indicate an increased risk of pelvic organ prolapse in the immediate postpartum period. Rather,

available data show development of prolapse remote from vaginal delivery.

Although operative vaginal delivery is a known risk factor for obstetric anal sphincter injury and associated fecal incontinence, vaginal delivery itself has not been demonstrated to increase this risk. No data exists regarding the association between vaginal delivery and levator spasms.

Barber EL, Lundsberg LS, Belanger K, Pettker CM, Funai EF, Illuzzi JL. Indications contributing to the increasing cesarean delivery rate. Obstet Gynecol 2011;118:29–38.

Burgio KL, Zyczynski H, Locher JL, Richter HE, Redden DT, Wright KC. Urinary incontinence in the 12-month postpartum period. Obstet Gynecol 2003;102:1291–8.

Handa VL, Blomquist JL, Knoepp LR, Hoskey KA, McDermott KC, Munoz A. Pelvic floor disorders 5–10 years after vaginal or cesarean childbirth. Obstet Gynecol 2011;118:777–84.

Hannah ME, Hannah WJ, Hodnett ED, Chalmers B, Kung R, Willan A, et al. Outcomes at 3 months after planned cesarean vs planned vaginal delivery for breech presentation at term: the international randomized Term Breech Trial. Term Breech Trial 3-Month Follow-up Collaborative Group. JAMA 2002;287:1822–31.

Hannah ME, Whyte H, Hannah WJ, Hewson S, Amankwah K, Cheng M, et al. Maternal outcomes at 2 years after planned cesarean section versus planned vaginal birth for breech presentation at term: the international randomized Term Breech Trial. Term Breech Trial Collaborative Group. Am J Obstet Gynecol 2004;191:917–27.

Larsson C, Kallen K, Andolf E. Cesarean section and risk of pelvic organ prolapse: a nested case–control study. Am J Obstet Gynecol 2009;200:243.e1–4.

Nelson RL, Furner SE, Westercamp M, Farquhar C. Cesarean delivery for the prevention of anal incontinence. Cochrane Database of Systematic Reviews 2010, Issue 2. Art. No.: CD006756. DOI: 10.1002/14651858.CD006756.pub2.

Rortveit G, Hannestad YS, Daltveit AK, Hunskaar S. Age- and type-dependent effects of parity on urinary incontinence: the Norwegian EPINCONT study. Obstet Gynecol 2001;98:1004–10.

Sultan AH, Kamm MA, Hudson CN, Bartram CI. Third degree obstetric anal sphincter tears: risk factors and outcome of primary repair. BMJ 1994;308:887–91.

Wiklund I, Edman G, Andolf E. Cesarean section on maternal request: reasons for the request, self-estimated health, expectations, experience of birth and signs of depression among first-time mothers. Acta Obstet Gynecol Scand 2007;86:451–6.

4

Wound breakdown

A primiparous woman comes to your office 10 days postpartum after a forceps-assisted vaginal delivery with a third-degree tear. She reports increased perineal pain and bleeding. On examination, she is found to have complete breakdown of her wound with no evidence of infection (Fig. 4-1; see color plate). The most appropriate management strategy is to

(A) allow healing by secondary intention
(B) prescribe oral antibiotics and re-examine in 1 week
* (C) perform prompt surgical repair in the operating room
(D) perform closure in the office

Obstetric anal sphincter injuries occur in approximately 2.2–19% of deliveries in the United States. The few studies that have been done on complications of repair of such injuries are limited by their retrospective design. Perineal laceration breakdown is uncommon and occurs in only 3–7% of severe perineal tears. Most breakdowns occur within the first 2 weeks of delivery and are characterized by symptoms of increased pain, vaginal discharge, bleeding, and fever. Risk factors associated with wound dehiscence include smoking, forceps-assisted vaginal delivery, mediolateral episiotomy, increasing body mass index, and fourth-degree laceration. The strongest risk factor for subsequent breakdown is the interaction between forceps-assisted delivery and mediolateral episiotomy, which should be avoided if possible.

Breakdown of a severe perineal laceration can result in a large, open perineal wound that often is associated with soft tissue infection. Purulent exudate may cover the wound, and typically, numerous displaced sutures are present. If the rectal mucosa or anal sphincter is disrupted, the wound also may be contaminated with fecal material. In a survey of colorectal surgeons in the United Kingdom, the majority recommended a temporary fecal diversion based on their observation that most nonobstetric wounds of this size require this radical intervention. One case report recommends temporary ileostomy in a woman with breakdown of a fourth-degree tear; however, contemporary obstetric practice does not endorse this strategy because most obstetric wounds heal with preservation of the normal fecal stream.

No consensus exists on appropriate management strategies for wound dehiscence. A recent Cochrane review concluded that there is insufficient scientific evidence to make a recommendation. Historic surgical dictum was that delaying repair for a period of 3–6 months was required to reduce inflammation and promote revascularization. Expert opinion informed by evidence from retrospective studies, however, has evolved in recent decades from a strict policy of no immediate resuturing to that of an attempt at early surgical repair as soon as the infection has resolved.

When early postpartum perineal laceration breakdown occurs, three potential management strategies exist: 1) immediate debridement and resuturing after resolution of infection, 2) immediate debridement and healing by secondary intention, or 3) immediate debridement and delayed resuturing at 6 weeks to 3 months postpartum. The risk–benefit ratio of each strategy rests on the relative risk of repeat breakdown if an attempt at resuturing is made when the tissue is suboptimal versus the dramatic inconvenience and suffering of the woman living with an open wound for a prolonged period.

In the few studies that exist regarding attempted early resuturing, the intervention was successful and resulted in a significantly shorter duration of healing compared with delayed resuturing. Early resuturing is also far more acceptable to patients. The principal issue stressed by all investigators is confirmation that infection has resolved before any attempt at resuturing is made. Typically, immediate wound debridement is performed in either an inpatient or outpatient setting (depending on the degree of pain and soft tissue infection), and once the wound is adequately prepared, the resuturing is performed. Pink granulation tissue with no tissue induration, edema, or exudate must exist before resuturing is attempted. Antibiotics are required if deeper wound infection is evident.

Although comparative outcomes have been found for preparation of wound dehiscence through superficial debridement in outpatient care compared with inpatient care, resuturing of the wound cannot be performed adequately in an office setting. Sufficient light, anesthesia, surgical instruments, and retraction are necessary to facilitate anatomic closure. As intraoperative intravenous antibiotics have been found to reduce the rate of primary breakdown of obstetric anal sphincter tears, it is reasonable to recommend intraoperative antibiotics for secondary repair. Appropriate postoperative care includes a bowel regimen that facilitates the easy evacuation of stool. Figure 4-2 and Figure 4-3 (see color plates) depict this patient's breakdown after it was debrided and repaired.

Hankins GD, Hauth JC, Gilstrap LC 3rd, Hammond TL, Yeomans ER, Snyder RR. Early repair of episiotomy dehiscence. Obstet Gynecol 1990;75:48–51.

Hauth JC, Gilstrap LC 3rd, Ward SC, Hankins GD. Early repair of an external sphincter ani muscle and rectal mucosal dehiscence. Obstet Gynecol 1986;67:806–9.

Stock L, Basham E, Gossett DR, Lewicky-Gaupp C. Factors associated with wound complications in women with obstetric anal sphincter injuries (OASIS). Am J Obstet Gynecol 2013;208:327.e1–6.

5

Risk factors for obstetric laceration

A 35-year-old obese Hispanic woman had a second stage of labor that was 3 hours in duration. Her infant was in the persistent occiput posterior position. She underwent a forceps-assisted vaginal delivery with midline episiotomy. On delivery, the infant weighed 3,856 g (8.5 lb). The greatest risk of anal sphincter injury during this delivery was

        (A) midline episiotomy
*   (B) forceps-assisted delivery
        (C) infant weight
        (D) persistent occiput posterior position
        (E) Hispanic ethnicity

Obstetric anal sphincter injuries are documented in approximately 2.2–19% of vaginal deliveries and recent population-based studies in Scandinavia and the United Kingdom have reported increasing prevalence rates. Between 2000 and 2011, rates of third- and fourth-degree tears tripled in England. The wide disparity in global prevalence rates likely reflects differences in methods of detection and in rates of operative vaginal delivery. Anal sphincter injury is a known contributor to the development of fecal incontinence in women. Therefore, knowledge of risk factors is vital, as is the effort to reduce exposure to modifiable risk factors. A recent population-based study found that almost 60% of all women diagnosed with an anal sphincter tear had one or more modifiable risk factors.

Large retrospective cohort studies have identified the following primary nonmodifiable risk factors: primiparity, Asian or Hispanic descent, advancing maternal age, and higher infant birth weight. Women older than 25 years are reported to have twice the rate of such injuries compared with teenagers. The major modifiable risk factors are forceps-assisted delivery, vacuum extraction, prolonged second stage of labor, and midline episiotomy. Whether mediolateral episiotomy and epidural anesthesia play a role in obstetric anal sphincter injury is unclear. Higher maternal body mass index has been associated with a reduced risk of such injuries in several studies.

Mode of delivery is the key determinant of the risk of severe perineal tears. Large studies consistently have demonstrated that women with instrumental deliveries have higher rates of third- and fourth-degree tears. Several studies have evaluated the differential effect of forceps-assisted versus vacuum-assisted vaginal delivery. Forceps-assisted delivery is associated with a 1.5–4-fold higher risk of obstetric anal sphincter injury than vacuum-assisted delivery. In the United Kingdom, the use of forceps among all vaginal deliveries doubled between 2000 and 2011 and was associated with almost a threefold increased rate of third- and fourth-degree tears. Compared with spontaneous vaginal delivery, the risk of having an obstetric anal sphincter injury has been reported to be 1.5–14 times higher with forceps-assisted delivery and 1.5–4 times higher with vacuum-assisted delivery.

A significant interaction between mode of delivery and other obstetric variables may cloud interpretation of the data. For example, a large Danish population-based study recently reported that when a concomitant mediolateral episiotomy was performed with vacuum extraction, there was a significantly lower chance of obstetric anal sphincter injury. There was no protective effect of mediolateral episiotomy when used without vacuum extraction. Similarly, mediolateral episiotomy was found to be protective against obstetric anal sphincter injury in forceps-assisted and vacuum-assisted deliveries in the United Kingdom.

Fetal head position at delivery has been associated with risk of severe perineal injury. Several studies have reported that persistent occiput posterior position has a twofold higher risk of obstetric anal sphincter injury than occiput anterior. Early recognition of occiput posterior position could influence obstetric management to try to facilitate head rotation. Another modifiable obstetric intervention is maternal position at delivery; lithotomy and squatting birth positions have been associated with a twofold increased risk of obstetric anal sphincter injury. No increased risk was reported with either a kneeling or sitting upright position.

Altman D, Ragnar I, Ekstrom A, Tyden T, Olsson SE. Anal sphincter lacerations and upright delivery postures—a risk analysis from a randomized controlled trial. Int Urogynecol J Pelvic Floor Dysfunct 2007;18:141–6.

Gurol-Urganci I, Cromwell DA, Edozien LC, Mahmood TA, Adams EJ, Richmond DH, et al. Third- and fourth-degree perineal tears among primiparous women in England between 2000 and 2012: time trends and risk factors. BJOG 2013;120:1516–25.

Jango H, Langhoff-Roos J, Rosthoj S, Sakse A. Modifiable risk factors of obstetric anal sphincter injury in primiparous women: a population-based cohort study. Am J Obstet Gynecol 2014;210:59.e1–6.

6

Aging and hormonal effects on the pelvic floor

A 71-year-old woman is referred to you for symptoms of urinary tract infection, which have improved after a 3-day course of antibiotics. Her dipstick urinalysis is positive for leukocyte esterase and negative for blood. Urine culture is positive for *Escherichia coli*. She has had three culture-proven urinary tract infections over the past 2 years. She recalls that she had one to two urinary tract infections while in her twenties. She is sexually active with one long-term partner. On pelvic examination, she has no structural abnormalities and has stage I pelvic organ support. The best next step in management is

      (A) computed tomography (CT) urography
      (B) antibiotic suppression
      (C) cystoscopy
*   (D) vaginal estrogen
      (E) renal ultrasonography

Estrogen receptors are present in the vagina, urethra, bladder, and pelvic floor musculature. The decrease in endogenous estrogen levels after menopause results in atrophic changes and dematuration of vulvovaginal epithelium; decreased blood flow to the vagina, urethra, clitoris, and perineum; and decreased muscle bulk in the pelvic floor muscles. Vaginal estrogen has been shown to increase the maturation index of vaginal epithelial cells, lower vaginal pH, and shift vaginal flora away from colonization with *Enterobacteriaceae*, which protect against urinary tract infection. Two randomized controlled trials found that vaginal estrogen reduced the incidence of urinary tract infections in postmenopausal women.

Recurrent urinary tract infections are defined as two or more infections in 6 months or three or more infections in 1 year. Despite this patient's bothersome symptoms, she does not meet the criteria for recurrence. Therefore, to prescribe daily suppressive antibiotic therapy would not be the best next step in her management.

It is common to use CT urography to evaluate for structural anomalies of the kidneys and ureters, nephrolithiasis, or upper urinary tract malignancy. The method comprises a triphasic study of imagery: images are taken 1) before intravenous administration of contrast to visualize radiopaque kidney stones, 2) during administration of contrast to visualize the kidneys and renal pelvis, and 3) after administration of contrast, allowing the kidneys to excrete the contrast, thus opacifying the ureters. The American Urological Association guidelines stress use of imaging with kidney or bladder ultrasonography or CT urography for patients who do not respond to treatment. This patient does not have a history of recurrent urinary tract infections and has no hematuria and, thus, CT urography is not the best next step.

Lower urinary tract evaluation with cystoscopy is indicated in patients with gross or microscopic hematuria to assess for bladder cancer. Patients who have frequent urinary tract infections after pelvic floor surgery, especially with mesh implants, warrant cystoscopic evaluation to assess for intravesical foreign body as a nidus of infection. Given that the described patient's history and clinical presentation does not raise suspicion for renal anomaly, nephrolithiasis, or hydronephrosis, renal ultrasonography would not be the best next step.

American Urological Association. Adult UTI. National medical student curriculum. Linthicum (MD): AUA; 2012. Available at: https://www.auanet.org/common/pdf/education/Adult-UTI.pdf. Retrieved August 31, 2015.

Mody L, Juthani-Mehta M. Urinary tract infections in older women: a clinical review. JAMA 2014;311:844–54.

Robinson D, Cardozo L. Estrogens and the lower urinary tract. Neurourol Urodyn 2011;30:754–7.

7

Pelvic organ prolapse quantification

A 71-year-old multiparous woman visits your office with a symptomatic vaginal bulge. She noticed the bulge after her total vaginal hysterectomy 2 years ago, and it has become progressively more bothersome. On examination, she has stage III pelvic organ prolapse. She has a total vaginal length of 10 cm, and her vaginal cuff protrudes past the hymen; however, it is not completely everted (Fig. 7-1; see color plate). The correct pelvic organ prolapse quantification (POP-Q) assessment for this patient is

(A)

-2	-2	-8
3	2	10
-1	-1	-10

(B)

-3	-3	-8
3	2	10
-3	-3	X

*(C)

+3	+6	+6
3	2	10
-1	+6	X

(D)

+3	+6	+6
3	2	10
-1	+6	+4

(E)

+3	+10	+10
3	2	10
+3	+10	X

Since 1996, the POP-Q system has been the international standard for describing pelvic organ support in women. The POP-Q assessment allows for a reproducible and reliable description of the support of the anterior, posterior, and apical vaginal segments using precise measurements to a fixed reference point (the hymen). It consists of nine defined points that describe the position (in centimeters) of the anterior and posterior vaginal walls, cervix or cuff, posterior fornix, genital hiatus, perineal body, and total vaginal length.

In Figure 7-2, the top row represents two points on the anterior vaginal wall and the vaginal apex. Point "Aa," or the urethrovesical crease, is defined as a midline point on the anterior vaginal wall 3 cm inside the hymen in a woman with no support deficits; "Ba" is the most prolapsed point on the anterior vaginal wall; and "C" represents the cervix or vaginal cuff in a woman with a prior total hysterectomy. The bottom row represents two points on the posterior vaginal wall, "Ap" and "Bp," corresponding to anterior vaginal wall points "Aa" and "Ba," and point "D," or the posterior fornix. Women with a prior total hysterectomy will not have a point "D". The anatomic position of these points is described in centimeters above or proximal to the hymen (negative number) or centimeters below or distal to the hymen (positive number) with the hymen defined as zero. The center row contains measurements in centimeters for the genital hiatus (external urethral meatus to hymen), the perineal body (hymen to midanal opening), and total vaginal length. The individual POP-Q points are combined to create a

Anterior wall **Aa**	Anterior wall **Ba**	Cervix or cuff **C**
Genital hiatus **gh**	Perineal body **pb**	Total vaginal length **tvl**
Posterior wall **Ap**	Posterior wall **Bp**	Posterior fornix **D**

FIG. 7-2. Pelvic organ prolapse quantification (POP-Q). (Bump RC, Mattiasson A, Bo K, Brubaker LP, DeLancey JO, Klarskov P, et al. The standardization of terminology of female pelvic organ prolapse and pelvic floor dysfunction. Am J Obstet Gynecol 1996;175:10–7.)

prolapse stage to describe the patient's overall condition, a total of five stages ranging from zero (no prolapse) to IV (complete eversion). In stage I prolapse, the criteria for stage 0 are not met, but the most prolapsed vaginal segment is more than 1 cm inside the hymen (less than −1). If the most distal or prolapsed portion of the vagina is within 1 cm of the hymen (inside or beyond), criteria for stage II are met. In stage III prolapse, the most pro-

lapsed portion of the vagina is more than 1 cm beyond the hymen, but not within 2 cm of the total vaginal length. In stage IV prolapse, the most prolapsed portion of the vagina is within 2 cm of the total vaginal length.

The described patient has undergone a prior total hysterectomy, so she would not have a posterior vaginal fornix or point "D," making options A and D incorrect. The POP-Q in option B is consistent with stage I pelvic organ prolapse. The vaginal apex or cuff is suspended 8 cm inside the hymen (C=−8), which is inconsistent with this patient's cuff extending beyond the hymen and stage III pelvic organ prolapse. Option C shows the correct POP-Q for the patient. It shows a 10 cm total vaginal length with the distal anterior vaginal wall and cuff located 6 cm beyond the hymen. Because the most prolapsed point is more than 1 cm outside the hymen, but not within 2 cm of the total vaginal length, her POP-Q describes stage III pelvic organ prolapse.

Option E is incorrect because the vagina is completely everted, with point "C" being 10 cm beyond the hymen in a patient with a total vaginal length of 10 cm. A patient with such a POP-Q would have stage IV pelvic organ prolapse.

Bump RC, Mattiasson A, Bo K, Brubaker LP, DeLancey JO, Klarskov P, et al. The standardization of terminology of female pelvic organ prolapse and pelvic floor dysfunction. Am J Obstet Gynecol 1996;175: 10–7.

8

Office evaluation of incontinence

A 54-year-old woman comes to your office with urinary incontinence that has worsened over the past year. She reports leaking with coughing, sneezing, or laughing (two to three times per day), which requires a minipad. She also notes rare incontinence associated with a feeling of urgency. She does not have any bulge symptoms or bowel concerns. A standing cough stress test is carried out, during which small drops of urine are seen leaking from her urethra when she coughs. Her pelvic organ prolapse quantification test results are as follows:

–2	–2	–6
4	3	10
–2	–2	–5

Her urethra is hypermobile with excursion from 10 degrees to 85 degrees with straining. After sending a urine sample for culture and sensitivity, the best next step in her evaluation is

      (A) wait for culture results
*   (B) obtain a postvoid residual urine volume
      (C) multichannel urodynamic testing
      (D) dynamic magnetic resonance imaging
      (E) midurethral sling surgery

Urinary incontinence comprises any involuntary leakage of urine. Stress urinary incontinence is involuntary leakage on effort or exertion, or on sneezing or coughing. Urgency urinary incontinence is involuntary leakage accompanied by or immediately preceded by urgency. A patient can have stress incontinence and urge incontinence at the same time. The office evaluation of urinary incontinence starts with a thorough medical history and physical examination. History taking should include asking about the duration, frequency, severity, and bother from urinary leaking. The type of leakage should be elicited with questions such as "Do you leak with laughing, coughing, or sneezing?" and "Do you leak with a feeling of urgency, which is a strong sensation of needing to go to the bathroom?" The amount and frequency of leakage can be gauged by asking how many times the patient leaks and how many pads she uses. Common validated questionnaires and tools that may be used include a 3-day voiding diary, the Urinary Distress Inventory scale of the Pelvic Floor Distress Inventory, and the Bladder or Urine scale of the Pelvic Floor Impact Questionnaire.

A urogynecologic examination should be performed. This includes a lumbar and sacral nerve examination and testing for bulbocavernosus and anal wink reflexes. The presence of prolapse should be evaluated. A cough stress test should be performed and the amount voided and postvoid residual urine volume recorded. Urethral hypermobility is assessed. Historically, this has been done by placing a swab into a patient's urethra so that the tip sits at the urethral–vesical junction. The location of the swab in relation to the horizon is measured at rest and with straining. Hypermobility is defined as excursion greater than 30 degrees. However, almost all women with stage II, stage III, and stage IV anterior vaginal wall prolapse demonstrate urethral hypermobility, making a formal swab test unnecessary in the setting of concurrent advanced prolapse.

After the basic office evaluation is performed, some surgeons elect to evaluate a patient with urodynamic testing. Urodynamic testing involves the placement of a bladder and rectal or vaginal catheter and allows the direct measurement of bladder and abdominal pressure, as well as a calculated measurement of true detrusor pressure. Such testing allows for evaluation of the storage and voiding functions of the bladder. Specifically, detrusor overactivity can be observed, urodynamic stress incontinence can be determined, and Valsalva leak point pressures identified. Urodynamic testing is an invasive procedure, with risk of patient discomfort and morbidity such as urinary tract infections.

The Value of Urodynamic Evaluation study was a randomized noninferiority trial that compared preoperative office evaluation with urodynamic testing or office evaluation in women who had uncomplicated demonstrable stress urinary incontinence and who desired surgical treatment. In women with uncomplicated, demonstrable stress urinary incontinence, preoperative office evaluation alone was not inferior to evaluation with urodynamic testing for outcomes at 1 year. Women had to report stress-predominant urinary incontinence and have a positive result on a provocative stress test, a normal postvoid residual volume, and an assessment of urethral mobility, with confirmation of the absence of bladder infection. If a preoperative workup is performed and within normal limits, then multichannel urodynamic testing is not necessary.

In the described patient with no prolapse and stress-predominant urinary incontinence, urodynamic testing could be avoided as long as the criteria set forth in the Value of Urodynamic Evaluation trial are met. She has demonstrated urinary leakage on examination and ure-

thral hypermobility. After urinalysis and urine culture are obtained, a normal postvoid residual urine volume should be documented to rule out urinary retention. After negative urine culture is confirmed, surgical treatment may be offered to the patient. Dynamic magnetic resonance imaging is not part of the standard workup for stress incontinence.

Abrams P, Cardozo L, Fall M, Griffiths D, Rosier P, Ulmsten U, et al. The standardisation of terminology in lower urinary tract function: report from the standardisation sub-committee of the International Continence Society. Standardisation Sub-Committee of the International Continence Society. Urology 2003;61:37–49.

Cogan SL, Weber AM, Hammel JP. Is urethral mobility really being assessed by the pelvic organ prolapse quantification (POP-Q) system? Obstet Gynecol 2002;99:473–6.

Nager CW, Brubaker L, Litman HJ, Zyczynski HM, Varner RE, Amundsen C, et al. A randomized trial of urodynamic testing before stress-incontinence surgery. Urinary Incontinence Treatment Network. N Engl J Med 2012;366:1987–97.

Urinary incontinence in women. ACOG Practice Bulletin No. 63. American College of Obstetricians and Gynecologists. Obstet Gynecol 2005;105:1533–45.

9

Urgency urinary incontinence

A 46-year-old woman, para 2, reports urinary incontinence that is intermittent throughout the day and night and has become more severe over the past 4 months. She describes leaking when running to the bathroom, after sneezing, and when getting out of the car after a long trip. She notes waking up once or twice at night with a strong desire to void and leaking on the way to the toilet. You elicit a medical history and perform multichannel cystometrography (Fig. 9-1; see color plate). The best next step in management is

    (A) incontinence ring pessary
    (B) periurethral bulking injection
*   (C) fluid intake modulation and timed voiding
    (D) pelvic floor physical therapy
    (E) trial of sacral neuromodulation

The described patient's symptoms and urodynamic findings of detrusor overactivity are consistent with urgency incontinence. The first-line approach to treatment of urgency incontinence is behavioral modification, such as modulation of amount and timing of fluid intake as well as timed voiding. Comparative studies have shown that consistent timed voiding reduces symptoms of urgency incontinence as much as anticholinergic medications without the adverse effects associated with anticholinergics, such as constipation, dry mouth, drowsiness, blurred vision, and sedation.

An incontinence ring pessary, periurethral bulking injection, and pelvic floor physical therapy are modalities used in the treatment of stress urinary incontinence. Such methods are less likely to alleviate this patient's urgency incontinence symptoms.

Sacral neuromodulation has been found to be effective in the treatment of urgency incontinence. It involves the placement of a stimulator lead into the S2 nerve root. If there is significant improvement of urgency incontinence symptoms during the trial period, a permanent neurostimulator and battery are implanted, typically into the adipose layer in the upper buttock. Explantation due to surgical site infection, lead displacement, and battery migration are not uncommon. Before a trial of sacral neuromodulation, a patient should be offered more conservative treatments for urgency incontinence, such as behavioral modification, anticholinergics, intravesical botulinum-A toxin injection, or percutaneous tibial nerve stimulation, all of which have been shown to improve symptoms of urgency and urge incontinence.

Gormley EA, Lightner DJ, Burgio KL, Chai TC, Clemens JQ, Culkin DJ, et al. Diagnosis and treatment of overactive bladder (non-neurogenic) in adults: AUA/SUFU guidelines. Linthicum (MD): American Urological Association; 2014. Available at: http://www.auanet.org/common/pdf/education/clinical-guidance/Overactive-Bladder.pdf. Retrieved August 31, 2015.

Groen J, Blok BF, Bosch JL. Sacral neuromodulation as treatment for refractory idiopathic urge urinary incontinence: 5-year results of a longitudinal study in 60 women. J Urol 2011;186:954–9.

Richter HE, Burgio KL, Brubaker L, Nygaard IE, Ye W, Weidner A, et al. Continence pessary compared with behavioral therapy or combined therapy for stress incontinence: a randomized controlled trial. Pelvic Floor Disorders Network. Obstet Gynecol 2010;115:609–17.

Shamliyan T, Wyman J, Kane RL. Nonsurgical treatments for urinary incontinence in adult women: diagnosis and comparative effectiveness. Comparative effectiveness review no. 36. Rockville (MD): Agency for Healthcare Research and Quality; 2012. Available at: http://effective healthcare.ahrq.gov/ehc/products/169/834/urinary-incontinence-treatment-report-130909.pdf. Retrieved September 3, 2015.

10

Urinary incontinence treatment options

A 62-year-old obese woman has a diagnosis of mixed urinary incontinence after her workup. She does not want to undergo a surgical procedure but desires to try behavioral interventions. Along with pelvic floor muscle exercises, the intervention that is most likely to reduce leakage is

      (A) weighted vaginal cones
      (B) incontinence pessary
      (C) elimination of caffeine
*   (D) modest weight loss

Behavioral treatment options for urinary incontinence aim to improve bladder control by changing the patient's behavior and by teaching skills for preventing urine loss. Examples include bladder retraining with timed voiding, dietary changes with reduction in excessive fluid consumption, pelvic floor muscle training, biofeedback, and behavioral intervention programs aimed at weight loss. These interventions are effective in 55–85% of women and are not associated with any significant adverse effects. Treatment efficacy, however, is limited by the need for long-term adherence.

Several randomized trials have investigated the differential effect of variable behavioral interventions on urinary incontinence. In women with stress incontinence, pelvic floor muscle therapy was found to be superior to the use of a vaginal pessary, and there was no additional benefit to combination therapy with pessary and physical therapy. Only one third of women managed with a pessary reported success, whereas more than 50% of women who underwent pelvic floor muscle exercises were much improved. In women with stress incontinence, the use of

behavioral training alone was equal to that of pelvic floor electrical stimulation.

A randomized trial of a 6-month behavioral intervention program to target weight loss in overweight and obese women who had at least 10 urinary incontinence episodes per week reported a significant effect on urinary incontinence reduction compared with a structured education program alone. The women in the intervention group had a mean weight loss of 8% compared with 1.6% in the control group. After 6 months, the mean weekly number of incontinence episodes decreased by 47% in the intervention group, compared with 28% in the control group. The results of this study highlight the significant benefits of modest weight loss on all self-reported urinary incontinence episodes.

The association between caffeine consumption and urinary incontinence was investigated in women enrolled in the National Health and Nutrition Examination Survey. Although caffeine consumption in the highest quartile was weakly associated with any incontinence, there was no significant association in women with moderate-to-severe urinary incontinence. In the Nurses' Health Study, there was also a weak association of incident urgency incontinence among women with the highest caffeine intake compared with women who had the lowest caffeine intake. No scientific evidence has demonstrated a significant beneficial effect of caffeine elimination even though it is commonly recommended in clinical practice.

The use of weighted vaginal cones for urinary incontinence was investigated recently in a systematic review of 23 trials that included 1,800 women. Weighted vaginal cones were noted to be better than no active treatment in women with stress incontinence and may be of similar effectiveness for pelvic floor muscle training, but they do not offer any additional benefit compared with pelvic floor exercises alone.

Goode PS, Burgio KL, Locher JL, Roth DL, Umlauf MG, Richter HE, et al. Effect of behavioral training with or without pelvic floor electrical stimulation on stress incontinence in women: a randomized controlled trial. JAMA 2003;290:345–52.

Richter HE, Burgio KL, Brubaker L, Nygaard IE, Ye W, Weidner A, et al. Continence pessary compared with behavioral therapy or combined therapy for stress incontinence: a randomized controlled trial. Pelvic Floor Disorders Network. Obstet Gynecol 2010;115:609–17.

Subak LL, Wing R, West DS, Franklin F, Vittinghoff E, Creasman JM, et al. Weight loss to treat urinary incontinence in overweight and obese women. PRIDE Investigators. N Engl J Med 2009;360:481–90.

11

Stress urinary incontinence

A 32-year-old woman, gravida 1, para 1, comes to your clinic with urinary incontinence. She hopes to become pregnant within the next year. She reports that after delivery of her son 8 months ago, she developed urine leakage with exercise, and specifically with running. The leakage interferes with her quality of life. She has no symptoms of urgency urinary incontinence. The best treatment option for her is

*   (A) incontinence dish pessary
        (B) urethral bulking
        (C) bladder neck fascial sling
        (D) synthetic midurethral sling
        (E) anticholinergic medication

Stress urinary incontinence is defined as the involuntary loss of urine with effort or physical exertion or with sneezing or coughing that affects a woman's quality of life. Nearly 16% of women report symptoms of stress urinary incontinence, and among women who have the condition, approximately 78% report that their symptoms are bothersome. Approximately 29% of those women say their symptoms are moderately to extremely bothersome.

Pessaries are effective in many women for controlling stress urinary incontinence symptoms by supporting the urethra and increasing urethral resistance (Fig. 11-1; see color plate). Such pessaries come in multiple shapes and sizes, with incontinence rings and dishes being most common (Fig. 11-2; see color plate). In addition, some pessaries offer the benefit of controlling incontinence and prolapse symptoms by having a knob and floor for support (Fig. 11-3; see color plate). Pessaries often are effective temporizing devices for women who have not completed childbearing. A multicenter randomized trial to compare efficacy of behavioral therapy with pelvic floor muscle training, incontinence pessaries, and combination behavioral–physical therapy and incontinence pessaries in women with predominant stress urinary incontinence found that patient satisfaction was slightly higher in the behavioral–physical therapy group (75%) compared with the pessary group (63%) and that combination therapy was not markedly superior (79%); however, satisfaction decreased within a year in all groups to approximately 50%, with only one third of patients reporting their symptoms were "very much" or "much better." By 1 year, 27% of women who had been fitted successfully with a pessary stopped using the device.

Urethral bulking agents treat stress urinary incontinence by increasing coaptation of the urethra, thus increasing urethral resistance. Urethral bulking is an effective temporary treatment for stress urinary incontinence, although success rates are lower than those achieved with surgery. A recent Cochrane review concluded that there was insufficient evidence for urethral bulking to guide clinical practice; however, bulking agents still warrant discussion in the surgical management of stress urinary incontinence. Injectable therapy most often is reserved for women who wish to avoid surgery or women whose comorbidities preclude them from undergoing surgery. Given this patient's young age and plans for additional pregnancies, a pessary would be the best first-line treatment for her.

From 2000 to 2009, there was a 27% increase in the rate of surgical management of stress urinary incontinence, the majority of which was secondary to an increase in the number of sling procedures. Much of the increase in sling surgery is likely secondary to the widespread use of synthetic midurethral slings; however, bladder neck slings remain an effective treatment for stress urinary incontinence in select women. Several types of sling procedures are used to treat the problem in women patients. The procedures differ in the type of material used, location on the urethra, and the superior attachment point of the sling. The multicenter Stress Incontinence Surgical Treatment Efficacy Trial randomized 655 women to bladder neck fascial sling or Burch colposuspension and followed participants for 5 years. Patient satisfaction remained high (83%) 5 years after surgery. Minimally invasive midurethral slings are considered the standard of care for women who undergo surgical treatment of stress urinary incontinence secondary to their high efficacy, quick recovery, and decreased complications compared with bladder neck slings. The Trial of Mid-Urethral Slings compared retropubic with transobturator slings with satisfaction rates of more than 80% at 2 years after surgery. Few data exist to guide patients and surgeons in regard to the effect of future pregnancies or deliveries on successful sling surgery, so conservative therapies should be offered first in reproductive-aged women who desire future childbearing.

Antimuscarinic medications are effective for the treatment of urgency urinary incontinence, but not for the treatment of stress urinary incontinence. A recent systematic review found strong evidence that use of antimuscarinic medications results in clinical improvement and higher continence rates compared with placebo for reducing urgency incontinence. However, the medications are associated with significant discontinuation rates because of bothersome adverse effects. Overall, fewer than 200 women per 1,000 treated with medications achieved continence. Dry mouth was the most frequently reported adverse event.

Albo ME, Richter HE, Brubaker L, Norton P, Kraus SR, Zimmern PE, et al. Burch colposuspension versus fascial sling to reduce urinary stress incontinence. Urinary Incontinence Treatment Network. N Engl J Med 2007;356:2143–55.

Brubaker L, Richter HE, Norton PA, Albo M, Zyczynski HM, Chai TC, et al. 5-Year Continence Rates, Satisfaction and Adverse Events of Burch Urethropexy and Fascial Sling Surgery for Urinary Incontinence. Urinary Incontinence Treatment Network. J Urol 2012;187:1324–30.

Fultz NH, Burgio K, Diokno AC, Kinchen KS, Obenchain R, Bump RC. Burden of stress urinary incontinence for community-dwelling women. Am J Obstet Gynecol 2003;189:1275–82.

Jonsson Funk M, Levin PJ, Wu JM. Trends in the surgical management of stress urinary incontinence. Obstet Gynecol 2012;119:845–51.

Kirchin V, Page T, Keegan PE, Atiemo K, Cody JD, McClinton S. Urethral injection therapy for urinary incontinence in women. Cochrane Database of Systematic Reviews 2012, Issue 2. Art. No.: CD003881. DOI: 10.1002/14651858.CD003881.pub3.

Maher CF, O'Reilly BA, Dwyer PL, Carey MP, Cornish A, Schluter P. Pubovaginal sling versus transurethral Macroplastique for stress urinary incontinence and intrinsic sphincter deficiency: a prospective randomised controlled trial. BJOG 2005;112:797–801.

Nager CW, Brubaker L, Litman HJ, Zyczynski HM, Varner RE, Amundsen C, et al. A randomized trial of urodynamic testing before stress-incontinence surgery. Urinary Incontinence Treatment Network. N Engl J Med 2012;366:1987–97.

Nygaard I, Barber MD, Burgio KL, Kenton K, Meikle S, Schaffer J, et al. Prevalence of symptomatic pelvic floor disorders in US women. Pelvic Floor Disorders Network. JAMA 2008;300:1311–6.

Richter HE, Burgio KL, Brubaker L, Nygaard IE, Ye W, Weidner A, et al. Continence pessary compared with behavioral therapy or combined therapy for stress incontinence: a randomized controlled trial. Pelvic Floor Disorders Network. Obstet Gynecol 2010;115:609–17.

Shamliyan T, Wyman JF, Ramakrishnan R, Sainfort F, Kane RL. Benefits and harms of pharmacologic treatment for urinary incontinence in women: a systematic review. Ann Intern Med 2012;156: 861–74, W301–10.

12

Stress urinary incontinence

A 44-year-old woman, gravida 3, para 3, comes to your office and reports that she leaks urine with coughing, sneezing, and jogging. On examination, she has a positive cough stress test. She is interested in undergoing surgical treatment and recently heard about retropubic midurethral slings. You counsel her that the most common complication associated with a retropubic midurethral sling procedure is

      (A) bladder perforation
      (B) hemorrhage
      (C) neurologic symptoms
      (D) persistent voiding dysfunction
*   (E) urinary tract infection

Urinary incontinence is the most common pelvic floor disorder that affects women in the United States. The prevalence of urinary incontinence among U.S. women is approximately 16%. Stress urinary incontinence is the report of involuntary loss of urine on effort or physical exertion, or on sneezing or coughing. Clinical evaluation of patients with symptoms of stress urinary incontinence requires a complete physical examination, including an assessment of the vulva, urethra, vagina, uterus, adnexa, pelvic floor muscles, and rectum; a screening neurologic examination; a postvoid residual urine volume measurement; and urinalysis. The presence of stress incontinence should be demonstrated objectively with a positive cough stress test (visualization of urine loss from the urethra during a cough or Valsalva maneuver) or findings of urodynamic stress incontinence on multichannel urodynamics before any surgical intervention.

The historical standard for surgical treatment of stress urinary incontinence is a retropubic colposuspension, with the most common procedure being a modified Burch retropubic colposuspension (Fig. 12-1; see color plate). This procedure is traditionally performed via laparotomy and attaches the endopelvic fascia at the midurethra to proximal urethra to the bilateral pectineal (Cooper) ligaments. Another historically common procedure is the autologous fascial bladder neck sling (or pubovaginal sling). This surgery necessitates a small abdominal incision to harvest a graft of anterior rectus fascia, which is fashioned into a sling. A vaginal incision is made and the fascial sling is placed at the level of the proximal urethra and bladder neck, then tunneled bilaterally through the retropubic space and attached to the rectus fascia. In a large, multicenter, randomized clinical trial, the autologous rectus fascial sling was found to have higher success rates compared with Burch colposuspension but with higher rates of postoperative urinary tract infections, voiding difficulties, and urgency incontinence.

Synthetic midurethral slings, which were introduced in the 1990s, have become the most frequently used procedure in the treatment of stress urinary incontinence. They are as effective as Burch colposuspension and autologous fascial bladder neck slings but are associated with shorter operative times, quicker postoperative recovery, and fewer complications. The procedure involves making a small vaginal incision, placing a synthetic sling at the level of the midurethra, and tunneling the sling either through the retropubic or transobturator space. Unlike the rectus fascial sling, the synthetic sling is placed in a tension-free manner and typically is not anchored. The Trial of Mid-Urethral Slings randomized women with stress urinary incontinence to retropubic or transobturator slings. Using a composite primary outcome (negative cough stress test, negative pad test, no retreatment, no self-reported symptoms, and no leakage episodes on voiding diary), the procedures were found to be equivalent at 1 year. However, 5 years after surgery, treatment success for retropubic slings was 7.9% higher and did not meet criteria for equivalence. The most common perioperative complication of midurethral slings is a postoperative urinary tract infection, which can be associated with approximately 30% of cases. Although these infections should be treated appropriately, they do not seem to affect long-term outcomes.

Bladder perforation at the time of sling placement has been noted to occur approximately 5% of the time. When noted at the time of cystoscopy, the trocar may be replaced without any sequelae, and the perforation does not affect recovery time or surgical outcomes. Postoperative voiding dysfunction or urinary retention is seen after 3–45% of midurethral sling procedures, depending on the criteria used to diagnose retention; both adverse effects are more common after retropubic sling placement. Most often, the retention resolves with intermittent self-catheterization or indwelling catheter for a few days after surgery. Persistent urinary retention may require a sling release. In a randomized control trial, neurologic symptoms (numbness or weakness in the lower extremities) were more common after transobturator sling placement than retropubic placement (9.4% versus 4.0%). Other complications, such as vascular or hematologic events, are rare, with rates of less than 3%.

Albo ME, Richter HE, Brubaker L, Norton P, Kraus SR, Zimmern PE, et al. Burch colposuspension versus fascial sling to reduce urinary stress incontinence. Urinary Incontinence Treatment Network. N Engl J Med 2007;356:2143–55.

Evaluation of uncomplicated stress urinary incontinence in women before surgical treatment. Committee Opinion No. 603. American College of Obstetricians and Gynecologists. Obstet Gynecol 2014; 123:1403–7.

Ford AA, Rogerson L, Cody JD, Ogah J. Mid-urethral sling operations for stress urinary incontinence in women. Cochrane Database of Systematic Reviews 2015, Issue 7. Art. No.: CD006375. DOI: 10.1002/14651858.CD006375.pub3.

Haylen BT, de Ridder D, Freeman RM, Swift SE, Berghmans B, Lee J, et al. An International Urogynecological Association (IUGA)/International Continence Society (ICS) joint report on the terminology for female pelvic floor dysfunction. International Urogynecological Association; International Continence Society. Neurourol Urodyn 2010;29:4–20.

Kenton K, Stoddard AM, Zyczynski H, Albo M, Rickey L, Norton P, et al. 5-year longitudinal followup after Retropubic and transobturator mid urethral slings. J Urol 2015;193:203–10.

Richter HE, Albo ME, Zyczynski HM, Kenton K, Norton PA, Sirls LT, et al. Retropubic versus transobturator midurethral slings for stress incontinence. Urinary Incontinence Treatment Network. N Engl J Med 2010;362:2066–76.

Wu JM, Vaughan CP, Goode PS, Redden DT, Burgio KL, Richter HE, et al. Prevalence and trends of symptomatic pelvic floor disorders in U.S. women. Obstet Gynecol 2014;123:141–8.

13

Stress urinary incontinence

A 42-year-old woman visits your clinic with urinary incontinence. She first developed urinary leakage with exercise, coughing, and sneezing after delivery of her first child. She has completed her family and desires surgical management. She does not report symptoms of urgency or urgency incontinence. She voids seven times per day, and has no prolapse or vaginal bulge. Her postvoid residual urine volume is 55 mL, and urine culture is negative. The most important test in the evaluation of this patient for surgery is

      (A) urodynamic testing
*   (B) cough stress test
      (C) ultrasonography
      (D) cystoscopy
      (E) computed tomography urography

The described patient has stress urinary incontinence, or the involuntary loss of urine with exertion (eg, activity, coughing, and sneezing), that is bothersome and affects her quality of life. Treatments for stress urinary incontinence range from conservative options, such as behavioral or physical therapy and pessaries, to surgical procedures. The most common surgical procedures are midurethral sling procedures; however, other options include bladder neck fascial slings, urethral bulking agents, and urethropexies. Women with persistent bothersome symptoms or who decline conservative treatments may opt for surgical management of their stress urinary incontinence. A recent trial randomized women with the condition to physical therapy or midurethral sling and allowed crossover between treatments if participants were not satisfied with their symptom control. Approximately 49% of women in the physical therapy group and 11% in the midurethral sling group crossed over to the alternative treatment. The initial midurethral sling procedure resulted in higher subjective and objective cure rates at 1 year than physical therapy.

All women who opt for surgical management of stress urinary incontinence should undergo preoperative evaluation. However, the evaluation may vary depending on whether the patient has uncomplicated or complicated stress urinary incontinence. Women have uncomplicated stress urinary incontinence if they have predominantly typical stress urinary incontinence symptoms, an uncomplicated medical history and pelvic examination, normal postvoid residual urine volume, negative urinalysis, and demonstration of leakage of urine with cough. Given that this patient has uncomplicated stress urinary incontinence (typical bothersome symptoms, no urinary urgency, no prolapse, a normal postvoid residual urine volume, and a negative urine culture), she does not need urodynamic testing. A cough stress test demonstrating fluid loss from the urethra with cough is adequate. The cough stress test can be done in several ways. Often, it is initially done in the supine position during the pelvic examination. However, if leakage is not seen, it needs to be repeated while the patient is standing. Cough stress test sensitivity is maximized in the standing position with a full bladder or at 300 mL bladder volume. Two randomized trials found that management of uncomplicated stress urinary incontinence based on urodynamic testing does not improve treatment outcomes after midurethral sling. One multicenter trial randomized women with uncomplicated stress urinary incontinence to a basic office assessment or office assessment plus urodynamic testing and found similar surgical treatment outcomes with a midurethral sling at 1 year.

Ultrasonography is not used in the evaluation of stress urinary incontinence. Although some investigators have described using ultrasonography to evaluate urethral hypermobility, this is not necessary in women who desire surgery for uncomplicated stress urinary incontinence. Cystoscopy is used to evaluate the bladder or lower urinary tract in patients with microscopic or gross hematuria, suspected mesh complications or urinary tract injury after pelvic surgery, or gynecologic malignancies involving the urinary tract.

Cystoscopy also may be used in the evaluation of urinary urgency or frequency and urgency incontinence in the absence of infection. It is not typically indicated in patients with uncomplicated stress urinary incontinence. Computed tomography urography is a triphasic computed tomography scan with and without contrast to evaluate the upper urinary tract in patients with suspected renal disease or upper tract abnormalities, including microscopic hematuria. Noncontrast phase is the criterion standard for diagnosing renal stones and is useful for evaluation of complex renal cysts and ureteral obstruction.

Dalpiaz O, Curti P. Role of perineal ultrasound in the evaluation of urinary stress incontinence and pelvic organ prolapse: a systematic review. Neurourol Urodyn 2006;25:301–6; discussion 307.

Evaluation of uncomplicated stress urinary incontinence in women before surgical treatment. Committee Opinion No. 603. American College of Obstetricians and Gynecologists. Obstet Gynecol 2014; 123:1403–7.

Labrie J, Berghmans BL, Fischer K, Milani AL, van der Wijk I, Smalbraak DJ, et al. Surgery versus physiotherapy for stress urinary incontinence. N Engl J Med 2013;369:1124–33.

Nager CW, Brubaker L, Litman HJ, Zyczynski HM, Varner RE, Amundsen C, et al. A randomized trial of urodynamic testing before stress-incontinence surgery. Urinary Incontinence Treatment Network. N Engl J Med 2012;366:1987–97.

van Leijsen SA, Kluivers KB, Mol BW, Hout J, Milani AL, Roovers JP, et al. Value of urodynamics before stress urinary incontinence surgery: a randomized controlled trial. Dutch Urogynecology Consortium. Obstet Gynecol 2013;121:999–1008.

14

Botulinum toxin for urgency urinary incontinence

A 55-year-old woman comes to your office with urgency incontinence. She states that she experiences five or six daily episodes of large-volume urine loss associated with an urge to void. She also reports enuresis with involuntary urination at night. She uses six to seven incontinence pads per day. She has tried behavioral therapy, including timed voiding and decreasing bladder irritants. She most recently tried two anticholinergic medications with no improvement in symptoms. She decides to try an intradetrusor injection of onabotulinumtoxinA. You counsel her that this is a very effective therapy but is accompanied by a high rate of urinary tract infections and the adverse effect of

    (A) dry eye
    (B) nausea
*   (C) urinary retention
    (D) leg weakness and numbness
    (E) psychosis

Urinary incontinence is defined as any involuntary leakage of urine. *Stress urinary incontinence* is defined as involuntary leakage on effort or exertion, or on sneezing or coughing. *Urgency urinary incontinence* is defined as involuntary leakage accompanied by or immediately preceded by urgency. Often, patients can have stress and urge incontinence. *Overactive bladder syndrome* is defined as urgency, with or without urge incontinence, usually with frequency and nocturia.

Initial treatment for urgency urinary incontinence is conservative and can consist of bladder retraining, such as timed voiding drills, urge inhibition, fluid restriction, and decreasing bladder irritants. Medication therapy with anticholinergics or β-agonists is another appropriate first-line treatment option. For patients with refractory overactive bladder syndrome (ie, who have failed conservative therapy, medication or anticholinergic therapy, or both), botulinum-A neurotoxin (botulinum-A toxin), peripheral tibial nerve stimulation, and sacral neuromodulation are treatment options.

Botulinum-A toxin is an effective treatment for patients with refractory overactive bladder syndrome. Botulinum-A toxin is injected with a cystoscope into the detrusor muscle with 10–20 separate injection sites (Fig. 14-1; see color plate).

In a double-blind, placebo-controlled, randomized trial involving women with idiopathic urgency urinary incontinence who were given either 100 units of botulinum-A toxin or anticholinergic treatment. The 100 units of botulinum-A toxin led to a reduction in urgency urinary incontinence episodes from 5.0 to 3.3 per day and to complete resolution of urgency urinary incontinence in approximately 27% of participants. Approximately 5% of participants were using a catheter at 2 months because of urinary retention, and 33% had a urinary tract infection.

These complications were significantly greater in the botulinum-A toxin group compared with the anticholinergic group.

Other treatments for refractory urgency incontinence include peripheral tibial nerve stimulation or sacral neuromodulation. Peripheral tibial nerve stimulation involves the placement of a needle electrode medially above the ankle to deliver electrical stimulation to the tibial nerve. In sacral nerve stimulation, electrodes are placed adjacent to the S3 dorsal sacral nerve roots and a pacemaker-like stimulator is placed under the skin of the buttock.

Dry eye is an adverse effect of anticholinergic medication treatment for overactive bladder syndrome, not of botulinum-A toxin. Nausea, leg weakness and numbness, and psychosis are not common adverse effects of botulinum-A toxin.

Abrams P, Cardozo L, Fall M, Griffiths D, Rosier P, Ulmsten U, et al. The standardisation of terminology in lower urinary tract function: report from the standardisation sub-committee of the International Continence Society. Standardisation Sub-Committee of the International Continence Society. Urology 2003;61:37–49.

Brubaker L, Richter HE, Visco A, Mahajan S, Nygaard I, Braun TM, et al. Refractory idiopathic urge urinary incontinence and botulinum A injection. Pelvic Floor Disorders Network. J Urol 2008;180:217–22.

Flynn MK, Amundsen CL, Perevich M, Liu F, Webster GD. Outcome of a randomized, double-blind, placebo controlled trial of botulinum A toxin for refractory overactive bladder. J Urol 2009;181:2608–15.

Sahai A, Khan MS, Dasgupta P. Efficacy of botulinum toxin-A for treating idiopathic detrusor overactivity: results from a single center, randomized, double-blind, placebo controlled trial. J Urol 2007;177: 2231–6.

Urinary incontinence in women. ACOG Practice Bulletin No. 63. American College of Obstetricians and Gynecologists. Obstet Gynecol 2005;105:1533–45.

Visco AG, Brubaker L, Richter HE, Nygaard I, Paraiso MF, Menefee SA, et al. Anticholinergic therapy vs. onabotulinumtoxina for urgency urinary incontinence. Pelvic Floor Disorders Network. N Engl J Med 2012;367:1803–13.

15

Urgency urinary incontinence

A 65-year-old woman has daily episodes of urgency urinary incontinence, despite the fact that she has reduced her fluid intake and performs Kegel exercises correctly. She requires one to two incontinence pads daily. She tried oxybutynin chloride three times a day with good success initially. However, she developed adverse effects (dry mouth, dry eyes, and constipation), which led her to stop using the medication. Her primary care provider is currently performing a workup for episodic hypertension. The next best step is to prescribe

    (A) mirabegron once daily
    (B) oxybutynin chloride XL once daily
    (C) oxybutynin XL twice daily
    (D) tolterodine tartrate twice daily

Antimuscarinic agents block the muscarinic receptors (M2 and M3) on the detrusor muscle, which prevents the binding of acetylcholine. In the bladder, M2 receptors are more common than M3 receptors (70–80% versus 20–30%). However, M3 receptors are thought to be most responsible for initiating bladder contractility. There are numerous anticholinergic agents available on the market today. Oxybutynin is a tertiary amine with M3 affinity, but it has some M1 affinity, which can result in central nervous system adverse effects. Oxybutynin also has direct myotropic relaxation and some local anesthesia. Tolterodine, fesoterodine fumarate, and solifenacin succinate are all tertiary amines that have M3 affinity. Fesoterodine is converted to its metabolite 5-hydroxymethyl tolterodine, potentially having fewer adverse effects. Trospium chloride is a quaternary amine that has limited penetration across the blood–brain barrier and, therefore, has the potential for fewer central nervous system effects. Oxybutynin also is available in a transdermal patch and as a topical gel.

The American Urological Association guidelines on overactive bladder therapy compared six different antimuscarinic medications. The investigators found no compelling evidence that one drug is better than the other when the reductions in daily episodes of baseline urgency urinary incontinence were compared. Across all medications, patients with worse urge incontinence at baseline achieved the most significant improvement, and patients with low baseline symptoms were more likely to experience complete symptomatic relief. However, these agents do vary in their adverse effect profiles. Anticholinergic agents are associated with significant adverse effects, including dry mouth, dry eyes, constipation, and blurred vision. Sustained release agents have more tolerable adverse effects than the immediate release agents. Despite the multiple agents available, the rate of discontinuation of anticholinergics is very high as a result of lack of efficacy and their adverse effects. Anticholinergic agents are contraindicated in patients with narrow angle glaucoma because these medications may precipitate an acute angle-closure attack.

For the described patient, tolterodine twice daily would not reduce adverse effects as much as a sustained-release anticholinergic agent. The best next option for her is to try a sustained-release medication, oxybutynin XL once daily. The dosage can be increased, but given that she responded well to standard dosage of the immediate-release agent, it is preferable for her to begin with standard dosage once daily.

Mirabegron is a β_3-agonist that relaxes the bladder by mimicking norepinephrine. Because β_3-receptors are predominant in the bladder, when norepinephrine is released by the sympathetic nervous system, it binds to the β_3-receptor, which causes bladder relaxation. Adverse effects of mirabegron include hypertension, nasopharyngitis, urinary tract infection, headache, and dry mouth, although to a much lower degree than anticholinergic agents. The only contraindication is uncontrolled hypertension, which may be exacerbated with mirabegron. Given that the described patient is undergoing a workup of episodic hypertension, it is unknown whether her blood pressure is controlled, and for this reason mirabegron is not the best choice for her at this time.

Gormley EA, Lightner DJ, Burgio KL, Chai TC, Clemens JQ, Culkin DJ, et al. Diagnosis and treatment of overactive bladder (non-neurogenic) in adults: AUA/SUFU guideline. American Urological Association, Society of Urodynamics, Female Pelvic Medicine & Urogenital Reconstruction. J Urol 2012;188:2455–63.

Sexton CC, Notte SM, Maroulis C, Dmochowski RR, Cardozo L, Subramanian D, et al. Persistence and adherence in the treatment of overactive bladder syndrome with anticholinergic therapy: a systematic review of the literature. Int J Clin Pract 2011;65:567–85.

Smith AL, Wein AJ. Urinary incontinence: pharmacotherapy options. Ann Med 2011;43:461–76.

16

Neuromodulation for urgency urinary incontinence

An 84-year-old woman visits your office with urgency urinary incontinence. She reports five to six daily episodes of large-volume urine loss associated with an urge to void. She wears multiple incontinence pads per day and feels unable to leave her house for long periods because of the need for frequent pad and clothing changes. She has tried behavioral therapy, including timed voiding and decreasing bladder irritants. She has narrow-angle glaucoma and is unable to tolerate anticholinergic medications. Her postvoid residual urine volume in the office is 200 mL. She has elected to pursue a trial of sacral neuromodulation. She had a permanent lead placed adjacent to the S3 dorsal root and is working on a daily bladder diary. Her diary today shows a greater than 50% improvement in her urinary leakage episodes. The most appropriate next step is to

(A) pull the lead
(B) replace the external battery pack
(C) acupuncture
* (D) place a permanent neurostimulator
(E) pursue percutaneous stimulation of the tibial nerve

Urgency urinary incontinence is defined as involuntary leakage accompanied by or immediately preceded by urgency. Often, patients can have stress and urge incontinence. Initial treatment for urgency urinary incontinence is conservative and can consist of bladder retraining such as timed voiding drills, urge inhibition, fluid restriction, and decreasing bladder irritants. Therapy with anticholinergics or β-agonists offers another appropriate first-line treatment option. For patients with refractory overactive bladder syndrome (ie, who have failed conservative therapy or medical or anticholinergic therapy), botulinum-A neurotoxin, peripheral tibial nerve stimulation, and sacral neuromodulation are treatment options.

Sacral neuromodulation is an effective treatment. There are two types of evaluation for sacral neuromodulation. A basic evaluation or peripheral nerve evaluation is performed in the office and involves the placement of a temporary lead along the S3 dorsal sacral nerve root, which is tested for up to 7 days. The advanced evaluation, or stage 1, is performed as an outpatient procedure. In the stage 1 procedure, the patient is placed in the prone position and a flexible lead with tines that anchor in place is aligned with the S3 dorsal sacral nerve root. This lead is stimulated with an external test stimulator and correct positioning is confirmed by observation of "bellowing" of the perineum, plantar flexion of the great toe, and the patient's report of sensation of tapping in the perineum. The lead is tested in the outpatient setting for up to 14 days. If adequate improvement is not demonstrated, the lead is removed in the operating room. The advanced evaluation has demonstrated better success rates compared with peripheral nerve evaluation.

Other possible treatments for urgency incontinence include peripheral tibial nerve stimulation and a botulinum-A toxin detrusor injection. Peripheral tibial nerve stimulation involves the placement of a needle electrode medially above the ankle to deliver electrical stimulation to the tibial nerve in 12 weekly sessions. Botulinum-A toxin is injected into the detrusor muscle above the trigone, leading to inhibition of calcium-mediated release of acetylcholine vesicles at the neuromuscular junction in peripheral nerve endings, which causes flaccid muscle paralysis and, thus, a decrease in detrusor contractions and overactivity. Because the described patient's bladder diary shows a better than 50% improvement in her urinary leakage episodes, she can proceed to stage 2, in which a permanent neurostimulator is placed. The lead should not be pulled and the external battery pack does not need to be replaced. Once it is determined that she has improved, a bladder diary should no longer be necessary. Acupuncture has not been shown to have proven efficacy to treat urgency urinary incontinence.

Abrams P, Cardozo L, Fall M, Griffiths D, Rosier P, Ulmsten U, et al. The standardisation of terminology in lower urinary tract function: report from the standardisation sub-committee of the International Continence Society. Standardisation Sub-Committee of the International Continence Society. Urology 2003;61:37–49.

Anger JT, Cameron AP, Madison R, Saigal C, Clemens JQ. Predictors of implantable pulse generator placement after sacral neuromodulation: who does better? Urologic Diseases in America Project. Neuromodulation 2014;17:381–4; discussion 384.

Kohli N, Patterson D. InterStim Therapy: a contemporary approach to overactive bladder. Rev Obstet Gynecol 2009;2:18–27.

Peters KM, Carrico DJ, Perez-Marrero RA, Khan AU, Wooldridge LS, Davis GL, et al. Randomized trial of percutaneous tibial nerve stimulation versus Sham efficacy in the treatment of overactive bladder syndrome: results from the SUmiT trial. J Urol 2010;183:1438–43.

Siegel SW, Catanzaro F, Dijkema HE, Elhilali MM, Fowler CJ, Gajewski JB, et al. Long-term results of a multicenter study on sacral nerve stimulation for treatment of urinary urge incontinence, urgency-frequency, and retention. Urology 2000;56:87–91.

Urinary incontinence in women. ACOG Practice Bulletin No. 63. American College of Obstetricians and Gynecologists. Obstet Gynecol 2005;105:1533–45.

17

Posthysterectomy fistula

A woman develops leakage per vagina on postoperative day 2 after a laparoscopic hysterectomy. Her surgery involved some intraoperative bleeding at the vaginal cuff, which was controlled with suture ligation, and she went home after she voided on postoperative day 1. She was prescribed oral phenazopyridine to confirm that the fluid was urine, and there was orange fluid on her pad. She underwent an office cystoscopy on postoperative day 3, which revealed a 0.5-cm × 0.5-cm defect in the bladder posterior to the trigone and 1 cm posterior to the trigone and medial to the right ureteral orifice. The best next step in management is

      (A) indwelling Foley catheter for 2–3 weeks
      (B) renal scan with furosemide
*   (C) computed tomography urography
      (D) immediate operative repair of fistula
      (E) renal ultrasonography

Leakage in the vagina after hysterectomy can be caused by urine from a urinary tract fistula (either vesicovaginal or ureterovaginal), peritoneal fluid, seroma, or vaginal discharge. Oral phenazopyridine will turn the urine orange and confirm a urinary fistula. When a vesicovaginal fistula occurs, an evaluation must be done to confirm there is no ureteral injury. Concomitant ureteral injuries occur in up to 12% of iatrogenic vesicovaginal fistulas. Upper tract imaging should involve complete delineation of the ureters. Hence, renal ultrasonography is inadequate because a ureterovaginal fistula may drain well enough through the vagina so that no hydronephrosis develops. Options for upper tract imaging include computed tomography urography with delayed view through the ureters or bilateral retrograde pyelography, often performed at the time of diagnostic cystoscopy. If there is a partial ureteral injury, such as a leak but not a total transection or ligation of the ureter, a stent can be placed at the time of the retrograde pyelography. In many cases, a stent will allow healing of the ureteral injury without the need for surgery.

Immediate operative repair of the fistula is not the best next step in management for the described patient for two reasons. First, it is not yet known whether there is an upper urinary tract injury and what operation would best address such an injury. Second, when a fistula is discovered, there is usually a significant amount of edema and swelling at the operative site. In the case of a nonradiated patient, it is best to wait at least 6 weeks for inflammation to subside before operating, and for some patients, a wait of up to 3 months is needed. In patients who have received radiation, longer delays are required. For small fistulas, use of an indwelling Foley catheter for 2–3 weeks is reasonable. However, for this patient, the important issue is identification of a concomitant ureteral injury, so use of a Foley catheter would not be the best next step in her management. A renal scan with furosemide will identify whether or not hydronephrosis is due to functional obstruction and would not be indicated for this patient.

Goodwin WE, Scardino PT. Vesicovaginal and ureterovaginal fistulas: a summary of 25 years of experience. J Urol 1980;123:370–4.

Rovner ES. Urinary tract fistulae. In: Wein AJ, Kavoussi LR, Novick AC, Partin AW, Peters CA, editors. Campbell–Walsh urology. 10th ed. Philadelphia (PA): Elsevier Saunders; 2012. p. 2223–61.

18

Surgical proctoring

As part of the hospital credentialing requirements, each surgeon must perform two proctored surgical cases. Your chairman requests that you serve as a surgical proctor for a new physician in the process of obtaining privileges. A surgical proctor would not be expected to

* (A) receive institutional compensation for proctoring
* * (B) teach a new faculty surgeon certain portions of the procedure
* (C) complete written evaluation of the new faculty surgeon
* (D) recommend termination of the procedure if the patient is at risk

Many hospitals have established surgical proctoring programs to credential new surgeons joining their staff or to credential staff surgeons on new procedures. The purpose of surgical proctoring is to ensure patient safety and quality of care by allowing the hospital to oversee and standardize surgical privileging. Because surgical proctoring plays an increasing role in hospital credentialing processes, it is important for urogynecologic surgeons to understand the role and expectations of a surgical proctor and how they differ from those of a surgical preceptor.

Surgical proctoring is meant to be part of a peer-review process to ensure that the surgeon can perform a procedure safely and competently. Therefore, a surgical proctor is meant to work on behalf of the hospital to observe and evaluate the cognitive and technical skills of the surgeon being proctored. The surgical proctor should not participate directly in the patient's care or see and evaluate her before the case. Upon completion of the case, the surgical proctor should complete a standardized evaluation form (provided by the sponsoring institution's credentialing committee) assessing the surgeon's performance and providing final recommendations regarding privileging on the procedure. To minimize conflicts of interest, the credentialing committee should identify surgical proctors for applicant surgeons; some organizations even recommend that the hospital compensate surgical proctors to minimize conflicts associated with industry overseeing and providing surgical proctors.

Technically, a surgeon serving as a proctor is not responsible for assisting or intervening in a case if a complication occurs. However, most experts believe that a proctoring surgeon should recommend that the procedure be terminated or at least intervene in the procedure if a patient is likely to be harmed. If the proctoring surgeon does intervene, he or she should be protected under a Good Samaritan law. The institution should indemnify the surgical proctor if he or she needs to intervene for the patient's safety. Any surgeon who acts as a surgical proctor should verify the indemnification with the institution before participating in a case. Some recommendations include having the patient sign a special consent form that recognizes that the surgeon is being proctored. The consent also should state that the surgical proctor does not have a preexisting patient–physician relationship with the patient and should verify the hospital's specific policy on intervention by the surgical proctor if a complication should arise.

In contrast, a surgical preceptor is someone who agrees to teach another surgeon how to perform a new surgical procedure. The surgical preceptor is involved directly in the patient's care and is responsible for the actions of the surgeon who he or she is precepting.

Heit M. Surgical proctoring for gynecologic surgery. Obstet Gynecol 2014;123:349–52.

Livingston EH, Harwell JD. The medicolegal aspects of proctoring. Am J Surg 2002;184:26–30.

Satava RM. Proctors, preceptors, and laparoscopic surgery. The role of "proctor" in the surgical credentialing process. Surg Endosc 1993;7:283–4.

Zorn KC, Gautam G, Shalhav AL, Clayman RV, Ahlering TE, Albala DM, et al. Training, credentialing, proctoring and medicolegal risks of robotic urological surgery: recommendations of the society of urologic robotic surgeons. J Urol 2009;182:1126–32.

19

Intraoperative cystoscopy

A 77-year-old woman, para 4, is undergoing vaginal hysterectomy and bilateral salpingo-oophorectomy with uterosacral ligament suspension for the treatment of stage 3 pelvic organ prolapse. You suspend the anterior and posterior vaginal cuff to the uterosacral ligaments bilaterally using delayed absorbable suture. After administering intravenous (IV) dye, you perform cystoscopy and fail to see urine efflux from either the left or right ureteral orifice. The best next step in management is

* (A) administer an IV fluid bolus
  (B) administer IV furosemide
  (C) insert open-ended stents
  (D) remove the uterosacral suspension sutures

In a study that used universal intraoperative cystoscopy, the rate of ureteral obstruction after a vaginal uterosacral ligament suspension was shown to be as high as 11%. However, with a bilateral absence of urine efflux, prerenal causes of oliguria in the described patient must be considered and addressed.

In a patient with no cardiac contraindications, an IV fluid bolus can increase urine output and expedite visualization of ureteral efflux on cystoscopy. Administration of a diuretic, such as IV furosemide, especially in diuretic-dependent patients, also can lead to more rapid visualization of ureteral efflux in the absence of a ureteral obstruction. However, it is not as easily available nor as innocuous as a fluid bolus and, therefore, would not be the best first step.

Tight packing with laparotomy sponges can compress the ureters and slow or prevent peristalsis, as can high intra-abdominal insufflation pressures during laparoscopy. It would not be appropriate to secure the uterosacral sutures without visualizing ureteral efflux. Although most cases of ureteral obstruction from uterosacral ligament suspensions are caused by kinking of the ureter, sometimes the stitch passes through the ureter, and leaving it in place will lead to a ureterovaginal fistula. Loosely tying the suture will leave a suture bridge, diminishing the effectiveness and durability of the suspension.

It should not be assumed that removing the uterosacral stitches alone will correct the problem. It is possible that the ureter was ligated or transected during the hysterectomy portion of the procedure. The cause of no efflux in this patient must be identified and corrected. Universal intraoperative cystoscopy at the time of gynecologic surgery has been shown to identify a substantial number of otherwise occult injuries to the urinary tract, thus preventing major long-term sequelae.

If removal of the uterosacral suspension sutures does not result in ureteral efflux, further investigations of ureteral integrity are needed. Catheterizing the ureteral orifice and passing a stent can provide reassurance about the patency of the ureter. Depending on the difficulty of stent passage, the stent may be left in place in order to minimize the risk of ureteral stricture.

Barber MD, Visco AG, Weidner AC, Amundsen CL, Bump RC. Bilateral uterosacral ligament vaginal vault suspension with site-specific endopelvic fascia defect repair for treatment of pelvic organ prolapse. Am J Obstet Gynecol 2000;183:1402–10; discussion 1410–1.

Gilmour DT, Das S, Flowerdew G. Rates of urinary tract injury from gynecologic surgery and the role of intraoperative cystoscopy. Obstet Gynecol 2006;107:1366–72.

Shull BL, Bachofen C, Coates KW, Kuehl TJ. A transvaginal approach to repair of apical and other associated sites of pelvic organ prolapse with uterosacral ligaments. Am J Obstet Gynecol 2000;183:1365–73; discussion 1373–4.

Visco AG, Taber KH, Weidner AC, Barber MD, Myers ER. Cost-effectiveness of universal cystoscopy to identify ureteral injury at hysterectomy. Obstet Gynecol 2001;97:685–92.

20

Pelvic organ prolapse

An 87-year-old multiparous woman with multiple medical comorbidities comes to your office for evaluation of pelvic organ prolapse noted during her recent hospitalization for myocardial infarction. She reports no typical prolapse symptoms but has urinary incontinence. On examination, her anterior vaginal wall is prolapsed 6 cm beyond the hymen, and her cervix is at the hymen. You obtain a postvoid residual urine volume, which is 260 mL. Urinalysis is negative for nitrites, leukocytes, and blood. The best next step in her management is

* (A) indwelling Foley catheter
  (B) antimuscarinic medication
* (C) prolapse reduction with pessary
  (D) urodynamic testing
  (E) colpocleisis and rectus fascial sling

The described patient has stage III pelvic organ prolapse, urinary incontinence, and urinary retention. Older women with advanced prolapse are at increased risk of urinary retention, which, in rare cases, may result in hydronephrosis. More commonly, retention may result in overflow incontinence and urinary tract infections. Because this patient has symptomatic urinary incontinence and is at risk of urosepsis, given her age and elevated postvoid residual urine volume, treatment of the urinary retention is warranted.

An indwelling Foley catheter is not a good option for this patient because it will not correct the underlying etiology for her retention and will increase her risk of developing a catheter-associated urinary tract infection, which is a leading cause of secondary health care-associated bacteremia. Patients experience an approximately 3–10% risk of bacteriuria per day of catheterization, and 10–25% of patients will develop symptomatic urinary tract infection. The described patient has multiple risk factors for catheter-associated urinary tract infection, including prolonged catheter duration, gender, age, and diabetes mellitus. Intermittent catheterization is associated with lower rates of bacteriuria and urinary tract infection than long-term indwelling catheters and is preferred over prolonged indwelling catheterization. If an indwelling catheter is selected, screening and treatment for asymptomatic bacteriuria is not indicated, and treatment should be based on urinary symptoms and fever.

Antimuscarinic medications commonly are recommended for treatment of urgency urinary incontinence. Antimuscarinic agents block parasympathetic muscarinic receptors and act on bladder M2 and M3 receptors to inhibit involuntary detrusor contractions. Their nonselectivity for muscarinic receptors in other parts of the body is responsible for the bothersome adverse effects associated with antimuscarinic medications such as urinary retention. Given this patient's elevated postvoid residual urine volume, antimuscarinic agents would be contraindicated and may increase her risk of urinary retention.

The patient's urinary incontinence may be from overflow, stress incontinence, or urgency incontinence. Overflow and urgency incontinence may be improved simply by treating the prolapse and elevated postvoid residual urine volume. A pessary is a good first-line treatment for women who are poor surgical candidates and have advanced prolapse and urinary incontinence. The described patient has multiple medical comorbidities and a recent myocardial infarction, making surgery a less desirable option. More than 90% of women with elevated postvoid residual urine volume will experience resolution of their urinary retention after their prolapse is corrected. One study showed evidence of bladder outlet obstruction in 72% of women with advanced anterior vaginal wall prolapse and who were undergoing urodynamic testing. Of these women, 94% had resolution of the obstruction after pessary placement. Nearly 80% of women with prolapse can be fitted successfully with a pessary. Multiple observational studies show that 70–90% of prolapse symptoms (ie, bulge and splinting), 40–50% of associated urinary symptoms (ie, stress and urgency incontinence and voiding difficulty), and up to 50% of bowel symptoms resolved with pessary use. Figure 20-1 (see color plate) shows a variety of different pessaries effective for treating prolapse.

Urodynamic testing is not indicated in this patient. Her primary pelvic floor concerns are prolapse and urinary retention. Initial treatment should be aimed at resolution of these issues. It is likely that her urinary incontinence symptoms will resolve with reduction of the prolapse using a pessary. Urodynamic testing is not necessary in the nonsurgical management of prolapse, incontinence, or both.

Colpocleisis is a safe, effective treatment for prolapse in older women. Compared with reconstructive procedures, colpocleisis is associated with shorter operative times, decreased morbidity, lower risk of prolapse recurrence, and high satisfaction. Case series demonstrate high retention resolution rates after colpocleisis in women with preoperative urinary retention. In a case series of 38 women with prolapse and urinary incontinence undergoing colpocleisis and midurethral sling, 11 women had preoperative retention. Out of the 11 women with preoperative retention, 10 had resolution of retention, and no woman experienced prolonged retention that required sling release. In contrast, rectus fascial sling is associated with a threefold increase in reoperation for postoperative retention when performed at the time of colpocleisis; therefore, colpocleisis with rectus fascial sling should not be performed in this patient. Figure 20-2 through Figure 20-8 (see color plates) show stage IV pelvic organ prolapse and the steps of colpocleisis.

Abbasy S, Kenton K. Obliterative procedures for pelvic organ prolapse. Clin Obstet Gynecol 2010;53:86–98.

Abbasy S, Lowenstein L, Pham T, Mueller ER, Kenton K, Brubaker L. Urinary retention is uncommon after colpocleisis with concomitant midurethral sling. Int Urogynecol J Pelvic Floor Dysfunct 2009;20:213–6.

Beverly CM, Walters MD, Weber AM, Piedmonte MR, Ballard LA. Prevalence of hydronephrosis in patients undergoing surgery for pelvic organ prolapse. Obstet Gynecol 1997;90:37–41.

Clemons JL, Aguilar VC, Tillinghast TA, Jackson ND, Myers DL. Patient satisfaction and changes in prolapse and urinary symptoms in women who were fitted successfully with a pessary for pelvic organ prolapse. Am J Obstet Gynecol 2004;190:1025–9.

Cundiff GW, Amundsen CL, Bent AE, Coates KW, Schaffer JI, Strohbehn K, et al. The PESSRI study: symptom relief outcomes of a randomized crossover trial of the ring and Gellhorn pessaries. Am J Obstet Gynecol 2007;196:405.e1–8.

FitzGerald MP, Brubaker L. Colpocleisis and urinary incontinence. Am J Obstet Gynecol 2003;189:1241–4.

Fitzgerald MP, Kulkarni N, Fenner D. Postoperative resolution of urinary retention in patients with advanced pelvic organ prolapse. Am J Obstet Gynecol 2000;183:1361–3; discussion 1363–4.

FitzGerald MP, Richter HE, Siddique S, Thompson P, Zyczynski H, Weber A. Colpocleisis: a review. Pelvic Floor Disorders Network. Int Urogynecol J Pelvic Floor Dysfunct 2006;17:261–71.

Leuck AM, Wright D, Ellingson L, Kraemer L, Kuskowski MA, Johnson JR. Complications of Foley catheters—Is infection the greatest risk? J Urol 2012;187:1662–6.

Robert M, Mainprize TC. Long-term assessment of the incontinence ring pessary for the treatment of stress incontinence. Int Urogynecol J Pelvic Floor Dysfunct 2002;13:326–9.

Romanzi LJ, Chaikin DC, Blaivas JG. The effect of genital prolapse on voiding. J Urol 1999;161:581–6.

Saint S. Clinical and economic consequences of nosocomial catheter-related bacteriuria. Am J Infect Control 2000;28:68–75.

Tambyah PA, Maki DG. Catheter-associated urinary tract infection is rarely symptomatic: a prospective study of 1,497 catheterized patients. Arch Intern Med 2000;160:678–82.

Weld KJ, Dmochowski RR. Effect of bladder management on urological complications in spinal cord injured patients. J Urol 2000;163:768–72.

21
Urinary retention

A healthy 35-year-old woman, para 2, comes to your office 6 weeks after uncomplicated placement of a retropubic midurethral sling. She reports urinary frequency, a slow dribbling urinary stream, and a sensation of incomplete bladder emptying. Her stress urinary incontinence symptoms have resolved after surgery. She reports no dysuria or hematuria. Her postvoid residual urine volume is 340 mL and her urine dipstick is negative. She is using self-catheterization. The most appropriate management of her condition is

        (A) trial of bethanechol
        (B) pelvic floor therapy
*   (C) surgical sling lysis
        (D) recheck postvoid residual urine volume after 6 weeks of self-catheterization
        (E) insertion of a suprapubic catheter

Midurethral slings are now the first-line procedure for stress urinary incontinence. Success rates range between 60% and 85%, depending on how success is defined and the length of follow-up. Urinary retention is a recognized complication of stress incontinence surgery; 30–45% of women fail the voiding trial performed on the day of surgery. The retention is most commonly transient and only 1.5–2.0% of women go on to require surgical sling lysis for persistent clinically relevant urinary retention after a midurethral sling. Severe retention typically is recognized within a few days of the procedure when the patient reports discomfort from an overly distended bladder. Less severe retention, characterized by chronically elevated postvoid residual urine volume, can present a diagnostic challenge. There is no absolute value of postvoid residual urine volume that is diagnostic or that excludes urinary retention. Instead, the act of contrasting the patient's preoperative and postoperative postvoid residual urine volume and eliciting symptoms of voiding dysfunction enable the diagnosis of iatrogenic urinary retention. If left uncorrected, urinary retention can lead to recurrent urinary tract infections, urgency–frequency, and urge incontinence. The described patient's symptoms and significantly elevated postvoid residual urine volume are reflective of clinically significant urinary retention that requires sling lysis in order to avoid the long-term sequelae of bladder outlet obstruction.

Bethanechol is a muscarinic medication that acts on the cholinergic receptors, mimicking the actions of acetylcholine. Muscarinic receptors in the bladder detrusor muscle are activated by parasympathetic signals from the pelvic nerve, causing bladder contraction and voiding. Bethanechol may be useful in patients who are unable to mount a strong detrusor contraction. It is highly unlikely that this neurologically intact patient developed detrusor hypotonia after a midurethral sling procedure. A pressure–flow study measures the detrusor pressure generated during voiding and the flow rate of the urinary stream. It can differentiate between a slow stream due to a hypotonic detrusor and a slow obstructed voiding pattern despite high detrusor pressures in patients with bladder outlet obstruction.

Pelvic floor physical therapy can be useful for scar tissue mobilization and can be employed as an option in the treatment of urinary retention after a pubovaginal sling (made of biologic materials) procedure. However, it is unlikely to loosen synthetic polypropylene mesh and, therefore, is not the best course of management.

Borderline elevations in postvoid residual urine volume and low-grade urinary retention can present a management challenge after anti-incontinence surgery. Postoperative patients have a variety of reasons to present with elevated postvoid residual urine volume in the immediate postoperative period, including postanesthetic effects, inflammation, tissue swelling, pain, and constipation. Most of these factors resolve within 2–3 weeks of surgery. The obstetrician–gynecologist should ask the patient with low-grade urinary retention to self-catheterize and measure the postvoid residual urine volume to see whether they normalize over time, obviating the need for an additional sling lysis surgery. This patient has substantially elevated postvoid residual urine volumes 6 weeks after surgery, and this is unlikely to change without surgical sling lysis. A suprapubic catheter is not going to resolve this patient's principal problem, which is a relative bladder outlet obstruction by the midurethral sling.

Brubaker L, Norton PA, Albo ME, Chai TC, Dandreo KJ, Lloyd KL, et al. Adverse events over two years after retropubic or transobturator midurethral sling surgery: findings from the Trial of Midurethral Slings (TOMUS) study. Urinary Incontinence Treatment Network. Am J Obstet Gynecol 2011;205:498.e1–6.

Glavind K, Glavind E. Treatment of prolonged voiding dysfunction after tension-free vaginal tape procedure. Acta Obstet Gynecol Scand 2007;86:357–60.

Rardin CR, Rosenblatt PL, Kohli N, Miklos JR, Heit M, Lucente VR. Release of tension-free vaginal tape for the treatment of refractory postoperative voiding dysfunction. Obstet Gynecol 2002;100:898–902.

22

Mesh complications

A 42-year-old woman reports urinary leaking with exercise, coughing, and sneezing after the delivery of her child 10 years ago. She has had no leakage associated with an urge to void. For the past few years, she has successfully used an incontinence dish, but she has decided that she is finished with childbearing and wants to pursue definitive surgical management. She underwent an uncomplicated transobturator midurethral polypropylene sling procedure. Cystoscopy at the time of the procedure revealed intact bladder and urethra with bilateral ureteral efflux. Six months after her sling surgery, she is happy that she can now exercise without leaking urine. However, she notes intermittent vaginal spotting between her menses and her partner describes "something scratchy" during intercourse. Figure 22-1 (see color plate) shows your findings on pelvic examination. You advise her that the most appropriate next step is

    (A) observation
*   (B) prescribe estrogen cream
    (C) surgically remove the entire sling
    (D) place a cadaver fascia sling over the existing sling

Initial treatment for stress urinary incontinence is conservative and can consist of bladder retraining, such as timed voiding drills, fluid restriction, and pelvic floor muscle strengthening. Other conservative options include incontinence pessaries, such as an incontinence dish or ring with a knob.

In terms of surgical options to treat stress incontinence, the midurethral sling has become the procedure of choice. It involves placement of a small synthetic mesh tape (usually polypropylene) vaginally, passing through the retropubic or obturator space. Complications after midurethral sling placement can include exposure or extrusion of mesh, voiding dysfunction, and pelvic pain or dyspareunia.

Mesh exposure is defined by the International Urogynecologic Association as displaying, revealing, exhibiting, or making accessible mesh (eg, vaginal mesh exposure). *Mesh extrusion* is defined as gradual passage of mesh out of a body structure or tissue. Often, the areas of exposed mesh correspond with the midline where the vaginal epithelium was closed intraoperatively or in the lateral fornices, especially if there is tension on the arms of the sling. First-line treatment of mesh erosion is estrogen

cream, which is the best next step for the described patient. If this is unsuccessful, small areas of mesh erosion can be excised in the operating room with mobilization of vaginal epithelial edges and direct closure with suture.

Voiding dysfunction can occur immediately postoperatively in up to 47% of cases. Voiding dysfunction is initially managed with intermittent self-catheterization or indwelling bladder catheter. Most of the time, this is a transient voiding dysfunction and the need for self-catheterization resolves over time. A small percentage of patients (less than 1%) require sling release in the operating room for persistent voiding dysfunction.

Pelvic pain and dyspareunia can result from sling placement, although they are more common after transobturator placement. Groin pain can be present with patient abduction or adduction, but such pain often resolves with time. Dyspareunia can occur from a tight sling or vaginal mesh exposure and often improves with sling release or resection. Recurrent stress urinary incontinence is possible after surgical resection.

Removal of the entire sling is associated with unnecessary morbidity and usually is not necessary for small, isolated mesh exposures. No definitive data exist to support the idea that use of a cadaver fascia sling placed over the existing sling would be an effective treatment. Because estrogen is a low-risk intervention, it is preferable to observation alone.

Abrams P, Cardozo L, Fall M, Griffiths D, Rosier P, Ulmsten U, et al. The standardisation of terminology in lower urinary tract function: report from the standardisation sub-committee of the International Continence Society. Standardisation Sub-Committee of the International Continence Society. Urology 2003;61:37–49.

Davila GW, Jijon A. Managing vaginal mesh exposure/erosions. Curr Opin Obstet Gynecol 2012;24:343–8.

Haylen BT, Freeman RM, Swift SE, Cosson M, Davila GW, Deprest J, et al. An International Urogynecological Association (IUGA)/ International Continence Society (ICS) joint terminology and classification of the complications related directly to the insertion of prostheses (meshes, implants, tapes) and grafts in female pelvic floor surgery. International Urogynecological Association, International Continence Society, and Joint IUGA/ICS Working Group on Complications Terminology. Neurourol Urodyn 2011;30:2–12.

Nazemi TM, Kobashi KC. Complications of grafts used in female pelvic floor reconstruction: mesh erosion and extrusion. Indian J Urol 2007;23:153–60.

Urinary incontinence in women. ACOG Practice Bulletin No. 63. American College of Obstetricians and Gynecologists. Obstet Gynecol 2005;105:1533–45.

23

Occult stress incontinence in patient with prolapse

A 65-year-old sexually active woman desires surgical management of her stage III pelvic organ prolapse. The vaginal bulge interferes with her daily activities, and she sometimes has difficulty emptying her bladder. She does not have symptoms of stress or urgency urinary incontinence. She experiences three episodes of nocturia each night. Her postvoid residual urine volume is 175 mL. She wants a procedure that will offer the best anatomic and functional outcome. The best next treatment for this patient is

* (A) sacrocolpopexy with Burch colposuspension
   (B) sacrocolpopexy without Burch colposuspension
   (C) colpocleisis with rectus fascial sling
   (D) colpocleisis without rectus fascial sling
   (E) sacrospinous ligament suspension with midurethral sling

The choice of route of apical prolapse repair should take into account the patient's goals and desires for surgery. Each procedure is associated with different inherent risks and benefits. The described patient is sexually active and desires the prolapse procedure with the best anatomic outcomes. A meta-analysis of three randomized trials involving 321 women compared sacrospinous ligament suspension with abdominal sacrocolpopexy. At 2-year follow-up, abdominal sacrocolpopexy was associated with significantly lower rates of recurrent vaginal vault prolapse compared with sacrospinous ligament suspension (4% versus 15% [relative risk, 0.2; 95% confidence interval, 0.07–0.8]). Likewise, sacrocolpopexy was associated with less dyspareunia than vaginal sacrospinous ligament suspension.

Approximately 40% of stress-continent women undergoing surgical repair of prolapse will develop symptoms of stress urinary incontinence after surgery. Therefore, many surgeons opt to perform a prophylactic continence procedure at the time of prolapse repair. For women with stage II or greater prolapse who are undergoing abdominal sacrocolpopexy, high-quality data support a concomitant Burch colposuspension rather than sacrocolpopexy alone.

The Colpopexy and Urinary Reduction Efforts trial randomized 322 stress-continent women undergoing sacrocolpopexy to concomitant Burch colposuspension or a control group with no Burch procedure. Burch colposuspension places two permanent sutures on either side of the midurethra and urethrovesical junction, then passes each suture through the Cooper ligament (iliopectineal line) to stabilize the urethrovesical junction (Fig. 23-1; see color plate). Three months after surgery, only 24% of the Burch group, compared with 44% of the control group, met one or more criteria for stress incontinence. Concomitant Burch colposuspension did not increase rates of serious adverse events or urinary urgency incontinence. Two years after surgery, only 32% of women who had a Burch colposuspension compared with 45% who did not (*P*=.026), reported symptoms of stress urinary incontinence, and there was a trend toward fewer urgency symptoms in the Burch group (32.0% versus 44.5% with no Burch colposuspension, *P*=.085). Based on the data that show lower rates of recurrent prolapse and dyspareunia after sacrocolpopexy combined with better urinary outcomes when a concomitant Burch colposuspension is done, sacrocolpopexy with Burch colposuspension is the best treatment for the described patient.

Colpocleisis is an effective, obliterative procedure used to treat apical prolapse in older women who are no longer sexually active. Rectus fascial sling is associated with a threefold increase in reoperation for postoperative urinary retention when performed at the time of colpocleisis. Neither colpocleisis with rectus fascial sling nor sacrospinous ligament suspension with midurethral sling is appropriate for this sexually active patient.

Sacrospinous ligament suspension is not the best treatment for the patient at this time because of her desire for an optimal anatomic outcome; however, a concomitant prophylactic midurethral sling at the time of vaginal prolapse repair should be considered. A multicenter randomized trial of stress-continent women who were undergoing vaginal surgery for anterior or apical prolapse found that 27% of women who underwent a concomitant midurethral sling, compared with 43% of those who did not have a midurethral sling, had stress urinary incontinence 1 year after surgery. Eight women in the control arm had surgery for stress incontinence in the first year compared with only one woman in the concomitant midurethral sling arm. Four women randomized to midurethral sling needed operative intervention to loosen the sling for prolonged voiding problems.

Brubaker L, Cundiff GW, Fine P, Nygaard I, Richter HE, Visco AG, et al. Abdominal sacrocolpopexy with Burch colposuspension to reduce urinary stress incontinence. Pelvic Floor Disorders Network. N Engl J Med 2006;354:1557–66.

Brubaker L, Nygaard I, Richter HE, Visco A, Weber AM, Cundiff GW, et al. Two-year outcomes after sacrocolpopexy with and without burch to prevent stress urinary incontinence. Obstet Gynecol 2008;112:49–55.

FitzGerald MP, Richter HE, Siddique S, Thompson P, Zyczynski H, Weber A. Colpocleisis: a review. Pelvic Floor Disorders Network. Int Urogynecol J Pelvic Floor Dysfunct 2006;17:261–71.

Maher C, Feiner B, Baessler K, Schmid C. Surgical management of pelvic organ prolapse in women. Cochrane Database of Systematic Reviews 2013, Issue 4. Art. No.: CD004014. DOI: 10.1002/14651858. CD004014.pub5.

Wei JT, Nygaard I, Richter HE, Nager CW, Barber MD, Kenton K, et al. A midurethral sling to reduce incontinence after vaginal prolapse repair. Pelvic Floor Disorders Network. N Engl J Med 2012;366:2358–67.

24

Painful bladder syndrome

A 57-year-old woman comes to your office with a 6-month history of urinary urgency and frequency plus bladder pain. She has been treated for recurrent urinary tract infections but reports negative urine cultures. On examination, she has pain with insertion of the speculum and bladder tenderness on bimanual examination. Otherwise, her pelvic examination is normal. Her urinalysis is negative. The most appropriate next step in management is

      (A) office cystoscopy
      (B) potassium sensitivity test
*   (C) pelvic floor physical therapy
      (D) pentosan polysulfate
      (E) amitriptyline

Painful bladder syndrome is defined as an unpleasant sensation (pain, pressure, or discomfort) perceived to be related to the urinary bladder, associated with lower urinary tract symptoms of more than 6 weeks in duration, in the absence of infection or other identifiable causes. The epidemiology of painful bladder syndrome is difficult to determine, given the lack of an objective marker to establish the presence of the condition. Studies rely on self-reported diagnoses, medical billing data, and symptom surveys. In a 2007 national phone interview study of 146,231 randomly selected households, the prevalence of painful bladder syndrome symptoms ranged from approximately 2.7% to 6.5% and affected 3.3–7.9 million women 18 years or older, depending on the criteria used for diagnosis.

Women with painful bladder syndrome have symptoms of urinary urgency and frequency with associated pelvic pain and possible dyspareunia. They may report a history of recurrent urinary tract infections, often with negative urine cultures and refractory to antibiotic therapy. Patients also may have a history of failed treatment for overactive bladder or endometriosis. The diagnosis often is associated with higher rates of depression, anxiety, sleep dysfunction, catastrophizing, stress, social functioning difficulties, and sexual difficulties. The pathogenesis is likely multifactorial. Current hypotheses include a defective urothelial barrier, autoimmune or infectious etiologies, and a systemic syndrome caused by central nervous system sensitization.

Given the lack of objective definitions of painful bladder syndrome, recommendations for treatment are difficult to establish. Furthermore, successful outcomes are limited. In a prospective longitudinal cohort study of 637 women with symptoms of painful bladder syndrome, overall symptom severity did not change significantly over 3 years despite the use of more than 100 treatment modalities.

The American Urological Association guidelines for the diagnosis and treatment of painful bladder syndrome provide a framework of recommendations. First-line treatment options, recommended for all patients, include education, self-care, and stress management practices. After these recommendations, the next line of therapy should include appropriate manual physical therapy techniques. Based on clinical principle, pelvic floor physical therapy may benefit patients with painful bladder syndrome and is without associated risks or adverse effects. A single-blind randomized controlled trial of 81 women with painful bladder syndrome that compared myofascial physical therapy with global therapeutic massage found a significantly higher response rate among those undergoing directed physical therapy (59% versus 26%). Amitriptyline and pentosan polysulfate are considered second-line oral agents for treatment of painful bladder syndrome. Both medications have demonstrated benefit in some studies but not in others; both also have adverse effects, including sedation, drowsiness, and nausea. As a result, use of amitriptyline or pentosan polysulfate is not recommended before attempting physical therapy.

Office cystoscopy used to be recommended for evaluation of painful bladder syndrome but is no longer recommended unless there exists a concern for calculi, bladder foreign body, carcinoma, or bladder diverticulum. A potassium sensitivity test also used to be recommended to evaluate painful bladder syndrome. The test involved instillation of a solution of potassium chloride into the bladder and evaluation of patient response as a diagnostic tool for painful bladder syndrome. However, given the low sensitivity and specificity of the test, it is no longer recommended.

Berry SH, Elliott MN, Suttorp M, Bogart LM, Stoto MA, Eggers P, et al. Prevalence of symptoms of bladder pain syndrome/interstitial cystitis among adult females in the United States. J Urol 2011;186: 540–4.

FitzGerald MP, Payne CK, Lukacz ES, Yang CC, Peters KM, Chai TC, et al. Randomized multicenter clinical trial of myofascial physical therapy in women with interstitial cystitis/painful bladder syndrome and pelvic floor tenderness. Interstitial Cystitis Collaborative Research Network. J Urol 2012;187:2113–8.

Hanno PM, Burks DA, Clemens JQ, Dmochowski RR, Erickson D, Fitzgerald MP, et al. AUA guideline for the diagnosis and treatment of interstitial cystitis/bladder pain syndrome. Interstitial Cystitis Guidelines Panel of the American Urological Association Education and Research, Inc. J Urol 2011;185:2162–70.

Hanno P, Dmochowski R. Status of international consensus on interstitial cystitis/bladder pain syndrome/painful bladder syndrome: 2008 snapshot. Neurourol Urodyn 2009;28:274–86.

Propert KJ, Schaeffer AJ, Brensinger CM, Kusek JW, Nyberg LM, Landis JR. A prospective study of interstitial cystitis: results of longitudinal followup of the interstitial cystitis data base cohort. The Interstitial Cystitis Data Base Study Group. J Urol 2000;163:1434–9.

25

Recurrent urinary tract infection

A 70-year-old woman with a history of chronic obstructive pulmonary disease has had recurrent urinary tract infections every 2 months for the past year. All of her urinary tract infections have been culture proved, and her symptoms have resolved each time with the use of antibiotics. She is not sexually active and has been taking vaginal estrogen for 6 months. She was given a prescription for once-daily trimethoprim–sulfamethoxazole but developed a resistant urinary tract infection after 3 months of therapy. Office-based cystoscopy is negative. Her urine appears cloudy, and she has a postvoid residual urine volume of 100 mL. After ruling out an active urinary tract infection, the best next treatment is

      (A) cranberry pills plus vitamin C
*   (B) methenamine hippurate plus vitamin C
      (C) nitrofurantoin monohydrate
      (D) increase vaginal estrogen to three times weekly

Prophylactic antibiotics are highly successful in preventing urinary tract infections among older adults, especially those who carry a postvoid residual urine volume. Daily nitrofurantoin is an ideal suppressive agent because it is excreted exclusively by the kidneys and is not absorbed into the gastrointestinal tract and, thus, has no effect on the gastrointestinal tract or vaginal flora. However, nitrofurantoin carries a rare but real risk of chronic interstitial lung disease in older adults and, therefore, would not be ideal in a patient with chronic obstructive pulmonary disease.

Methenamine salts have been shown to inhibit urinary tract infections by hydrolyzing in the urine (because of the acidity in the urine) into formaldehyde, which is bacteriostatic. As a result, there is no development of bacterial resistance to the medication. In order to optimize treatment and maximize urine acidity, methenamine is given together with vitamin C. Adverse effects include increased gastrointestinal acidity resulting in nausea or abdominal pain, as well as painful urination and gross hematuria. Methenamine plus vitamin C would provide the best next treatment alternative for the described patient who developed a resistant urinary tract infection after 3 months of therapy with trimethoprim–sulfamethoxazole.

At menopause, vaginal pH begins to increase, causing replacement of lactobacillus with pathogenic bacteria such as *Escherichia coli* and *Enterobacter*. This results in increased rates of urinary tract infections after menopause. In a randomized clinical trial, vaginal estrogen in the postmenopausal woman has been shown to significantly reduce urinary tract infections, from 6.0 to 0.5 infections per year. In a postmenopausal woman who has been taking vaginal estrogen, increasing from two times to three times a week is unlikely to cause a significant change.

The combination of cranberry tablets plus vitamin C has shown some efficacy in preventing urinary tract infections compared with placebo. However, a double-blind trial of 221 premenopausal women randomized to daily trimethoprim–sulfamethoxazole or cranberry capsules revealed better efficacy with prophylactic antibiotics. The mean number of urinary tract infections in 1 year was 4.0 (95% confidence interval, 2.3–5.6) in the cranberry group compared with 1.8 (confidence interval, 0.8–2.7) in the trimethoprim–sulfamethoxazole group. Cranberry juice, although popular as a supposed method for prevention of urinary tract infection, lacks proven efficacy.

Beerepoot MA, ter Riet G, Nys S, van der Wal WM, de Borgie CA, de Reijke TM, et al. Cranberries vs antibiotics to prevent urinary tract infections: a randomized double-blind noninferiority trial in premenopausal women. Arch Intern Med 2011;171:1270–8.

Dielubanza EJ, Schaeffer AJ. Urinary tract infections in women. Med Clin North Am 2011;95:27–41.

Madani Y, Mann B. Nitrofurantoin-induced lung disease and prophylaxis of urinary tract infections. Prim Care Respir J 2012;21:337–41.

26

Use of the POP-Q test to determine surgical options

A 63-year-old woman comes to your office with a vaginal bulge that she felt over the past year. She has had to push on this bulge to complete urination and defecation. She has no significant previous medical history and has never undergone surgery. She experienced menopause at age 51 years and has had no postmenopausal bleeding. She is sexually active. On examination, she has an intact sacral nerve. Her levator ani muscles are weak, with only a flicker of a squeeze felt on your fingers during examination. Her anterior vaginal wall reduces with support of the cervix with a large procto swab. Her uterus is small and mobile. Her pelvic organ prolapse quantification (POP-Q) test is as follows:

+3	+5	+6
4	3	10
−1	−1	+4

The best surgical option to correct her prolapse is

    (A) Burch colposuspension
    (B) anterior and posterior colporrhaphy
*   (C) abdominal sacrocolpopexy
    (D) vaginal hysterectomy
    (E) placement of vaginal mesh

Pelvic floor disorders, including pelvic organ prolapse, urinary dysfunction, and fecal incontinence, are common problems seen with increasing incidence as women age. The prevalence of pelvic organ prolapse stage II or greater increases to approximately 65% in women who are age 68 years. The etiology of pelvic organ prolapse is complex and involves potential injury to the many ligaments, muscles, and tissues, as well as innervation of the pelvis. Contributing factors include age, parity, abdominal circumference, and body mass index.

Many clinicians use the POP-Q test, in which the support defects of the vagina and perineum are measured systematically, including the anterior, posterior, and apical dimensions, along with the genital hiatus and perineal body measurements. The stages of prolapse using the POP-Q system are based on the leading edge of the prolapse. Stage 0 indicates no prolapse. Stage I is the most distal portion of the prolapse, at 1 cm or less proximal or distal to the hymenal plane. Stage III is the most distal portion of the prolapse that protrudes more than 1 cm below the hymen but protrudes no further than 2 cm less than the total vaginal length. In stage IV, vaginal eversion is essentially complete.

If performed efficiently, the ideal procedure will repair the patient's symptomatic pelvic floor defects, allow for rapid recovery, and comply with her sexual activity desires. The approach must take into consideration the patient's overall health, age, and physical activity status, and take into account previous attempts at repair.

Surgical techniques to address apical support defects include vaginal approaches and abdominal approaches, which can be performed through a traditional incision or a minimally invasive procedure. Vaginal approaches include uterosacral ligament suspension, sacrospinous fixation, and iliococcygeus fixation. These procedures can be done with a traditional native tissue and suture repair or with mesh augmentation. An obliterative option for those women who do not desire future sexual activity includes colpocleisis. Abdominal sacrocolpopexy involves the use of a synthetic polypropylene mesh and has a success rate of 76–100%, with a 4% reoperation rate for recurrent pelvic organ prolapse.

The described patient has no significant comorbidities; she has stage 3 apical prolapse and, thus, would benefit from an apical procedure, which is a long-lasting, durable repair. An abdominal sacrocolpopexy would achieve these goals.

A Burch colposuspension is a procedure to fix stress incontinence and, therefore, would not address this patient's apical prolapse. An anterior and posterior colporrhaphy would not address her apical defect and has a high failure rate. Similarly, a vaginal hysterectomy without an apical suspension would not address her apical defect.

Vaginal mesh is an option for the described patient but likely not the best choice in a young, sexually active woman. In 2011, the U.S. Food and Drug Administration issued a warning about serious complications associated with surgical mesh inserted by means of transvaginal placement to treat pelvic organ prolapse. The U.S. Food and Drug Administration warning stated that "serious complications associated with surgical mesh

for transvaginal repair of pelvic organ prolapse are not rare." Extra consideration is warranted in considering a patient's wishes for surgery and lifestyle before considering vaginal mesh repair for primary prolapse in young, sexually active women.

Nygaard IE, McCreery R, Brubaker L, Connolly A, Cundiff G, Weber AM, et al. Abdominal sacrocolpopexy: a comprehensive review. Pelvic Floor Disorders Network. Obstet Gynecol 2004;104:805–23.

Pelvic organ prolapse. ACOG Practice Bulletin No. 85. American College of Obstetricians and Gynecologists. Obstet Gynecol 2007; 110:717–29.

27

Mesh complications

A 63-year-old woman with anterior predominant pelvic organ prolapse comes to your office for a second opinion regarding surgery for pelvic organ prolapse. A surgeon has recommended an anterior colporrhaphy with synthetic mesh augmentation. She is considering proceeding with this surgery but would like to discuss possible complications associated with vaginal mesh. You inform her that the most likely complication after vaginal placement of synthetic mesh is

    (A) pelvic or vaginal pain
    (B) dyspareunia
    (C) recurrent prolapse
    (D) vaginal infection
*   (E) mesh exposure

In October 2008, the U.S. Food and Drug Administration (FDA) issued a "black box" warning on serious complications associated with surgical mesh placed through the vagina (ie, transvaginal placement) to treat pelvic organ prolapse. In a review of complications reported to the FDA in 2008–2010, frequently reported complications included mesh extrusion, pain, infection, bleeding, dyspareunia, organ perforation, urinary problems, recurrent prolapse, neuromuscular problems, vaginal scarring, and emotional problems. The FDA conducted a systematic review of the published scientific literature from 1996 to 2011 and found no evidence that the use of transvaginal mesh improved symptomatic results or quality of life outcomes over traditional repairs without mesh augmentation. The FDA noted that "erosion of mesh through the vagina is the most common and consistently reported mesh-related complication from transvaginal pelvic organ prolapse surgeries using mesh." The initial warning was modified in 2011 to specifically address mesh placed through the vagina for the purpose of correcting pelvic

organ prolapse without specifically addressing mesh used in the treatment of stress urinary incontinence.

Other studies have found similar outcomes. In a systematic review published in 2008, graft extrusion was noted to be the most frequently encountered complication (0–30%), followed by urinary tract infection (0–19%), visceral injury (1–4%), bleeding (0–3%), and fistula (1%). In 2011, the International Urogynecological Association, in cooperation with the International Continence Society, published guidelines for the standardization of terminology and classification for vaginal mesh-related complications (Fig. 27-1; see color plate).

Vaginal mesh complications may be treated conservatively with topical estrogen, antibiotics, or pelvic floor physical therapy, depending on the presenting symptoms. Often, however, surgical excision may be deemed appropriate if patients fail to respond to more conservative measures. Surgical excision does not guarantee complete symptom resolution. In a recently published retrospective analysis of 90 patients undergoing surgery for removal of transvaginal mesh, only 51% of patients reported resolution of presenting symptoms after surgical removal. Among these patients, the most common persistent symptom was pelvic or vaginal pain. Given the ongoing debate regarding use of vaginal mesh in the treatment of pelvic organ prolapse, it is imperative that health care providers follow FDA recommendations for use. These recommendations are listed in Box 27-1.

BOX 27-1

U.S. Food and Drug Administration Recommendations for Use of Vaginal Mesh

As stated in the October 20, 2008 Public Health Notification, the FDA continues to recommend that health care providers should

- obtain specialized training for each mesh placement technique and be aware of the risks of surgical mesh.
- be vigilant for potential adverse events from the mesh, especially erosion and infection.
- watch for complications associated with the tools used in transvaginal placement, especially bowel, bladder, and blood vessel perforations.
- inform patients that implantation of surgical mesh is permanent and that some complications associated with the implanted mesh may require additional surgery that may or may not correct the complication.
- inform patients about the potential for serious complications and their effect on quality of life, including pain during sexual intercourse, scarring, and narrowing of the vaginal wall in POP repair using surgical mesh.
- provide patients with a copy of the patient labeling from the surgical mesh manufacturer if available.

In addition, the FDA also recommends that health care providers should

- recognize that in most cases, POP can be treated successfully without mesh, thus avoiding the risk of mesh-related complications.
- choose mesh surgery only after weighing the risks and benefits of surgery with mesh versus all surgical and nonsurgical alternatives.
- consider the following factors before placing surgical mesh:
  — Surgical mesh is a permanent implant that may make future surgical repair more challenging.
  — A mesh procedure may put the patient at risk of requiring additional surgery or of the development of new complications.
  — Removal of mesh because of mesh complications may involve multiple surgeries and significantly impair the patient's quality of life.
  — Complete removal of mesh may not be possible and may not result in complete resolution of complications, including pain.
  — Mesh placed abdominally for POP repair may result in lower rates of mesh complications compared with transvaginal POP surgery with mesh.
- inform the patient about the benefits and risks of nonsurgical options, nonmesh surgery, surgical mesh placed abdominally, and the likely success of these alternatives compared with transvaginal surgery with mesh.
- notify the patient if mesh will be used in her POP surgery and provide the patient with information about the specific product used.
- ensure that the patient understands the postoperative risks and complications of mesh surgery as well as limited long-term outcomes data.

Abbreviations: FDA, U.S. Food and Drug Administration; POP, pelvic organ prolapse.

U.S. Food and Drug Administration. FDA Executive Summary: Surgical Mesh for Treatment of Women With Pelvic Organ Prolapse and Stress Urinary Incontinence, Obstetrics & Gynecological Devices Advisory Committee Meeting, September 8–9, 2011. Silver Spring (MD): FDA; 2011. Available at: http://www.fda.gov/downloads/UCM270402.pdf. Retrieved October 6, 2015.

Crosby EC, Abernethy M, Berger MB, DeLancey JO, Fenner DE, Morgan DM. Symptom resolution after operative management of complications from transvaginal mesh. Obstet Gynecol 2014;123:134–9.

Haylen BT, Freeman RM, Swift SE, Cosson M, Davila GW, Deprest J, et al. An International Urogynecological Association (IUGA)/ International Continence Society (ICS) joint terminology and classification of the complications related directly to the insertion of prostheses (meshes, implants, tapes) and grafts in female pelvic floor surgery. International Urogynecological Association, International Continence Society, and Joint IUGA/ICS Working Group on Complications Terminology. Neurourol Urodyn 2011;30:2–12.

Sung VW, Rogers RG, Schaffer JI, Balk EM, Uhlig K, Lau J, et al. Graft use in transvaginal pelvic organ prolapse repair: a systematic review. Society of Gynecologic Surgeons Systematic Review Group. Obstet Gynecol 2008;112:1131–42.

U.S. Food and Drug Administration. UPDATE on serious complications associated with transvaginal placement of surgical mesh for pelvic organ prolapse: FDA safety communication. Silver Spring (MD): FDA; 2011. Available at: http://www.fda.gov/MedicalDevices/Safety/AlertsandNotices/ucm262435.htm. Retrieved September 22, 2015.

U.S. Food and Drug Administration. FDA public health notification: Serious complications associated with transvaginal placement of surgical mesh in repair of pelvic organ prolapse and stress urinary incontinence. Silver Spring (MD): FDA; 2008. Available at: http://www.fda.gov/MedicalDevices/Safety/AlertsandNotices/PublicHealthNotifications/ucm061976.htm. Retrieved September 22, 2015.

Vaginal placement of synthetic mesh for pelvic organ prolapse. Committee Opinion No. 513. American College of Obstetricians and Gynecologists. Obstet Gynecol 2011;118:1459–64.

28

Apical prolapse

A 45-year-old woman comes to your office with symptomatic stage III pelvic organ prolapse. She has been using a pessary for the past 5 years, but now she desires surgical management. She is an avid triathlete, and she recently completed her first Ironman race. She does not report any urinary or bowel symptoms and is sexually active. Her apex and anterior vaginal wall are 5 cm outside the hymen. She desires the most durable repair with the quickest recovery time. The most appropriate surgical procedure for her is

    (A) sacrospinous ligament suspension
 * (B) laparoscopic sacrocolpopexy
    (C) uterosacral ligament suspension
    (D) colpocleisis
    (E) iliococcygeus suspension

Apical prolapse is the descent of the uterus, cervix, or vaginal vault and affects millions of women. Anterior or posterior vaginal wall prolapse without concomitant apical prolapse is uncommon. In fact, 77% of the size of anterior vaginal wall prolapse can be explained by the position of the apex and length of the vagina; therefore, apical prolapse repair should be included in most pelvic reconstructive surgeries.

The choice of surgical procedure or route for apical prolapse repair should be individualized and based on a woman's distinct goals for surgery weighed against the benefits, complications, durability, and recovery associated with each procedure. Historically, open abdominal procedures with synthetic mesh (sacrocolpopexy) are more effective at restoring vaginal topography, whereas native tissue vaginal repairs may be associated with less serious morbidity and quicker recovery. A meta-analysis of three randomized trials that compared open sacrocolpopexy with vaginal sacrospinous ligament suspension found sacrocolpopexy had lower rates of recurrent prolapse

(4% versus 15%) and reoperation (7% versus 16%) in the first 2 years. In another meta-analysis, total complication rates were similar for open abdominal and vaginal procedures (17% versus 15%); however, surgery through the abdominal route was associated with more complications involving surgical or radiologic intervention (6% versus 2%). Therefore, sacrospinous ligament suspension would not be the best choice in this active patient who desires the most durable repair.

Laparoscopic sacrocolpopexy is performed by securing the anterior and posterior vaginal walls via surgical mesh to the anterior longitudinal sacral ligament just below the sacral promontory (Fig. 28-1; see color plate). Sacrocolpopexy is more effective in restoring vaginal topography and may be more appropriate for women with risk factors for prolapse recurrence, such as young age, high-impact activity, obesity, advanced-stage prolapse, and prior prolapse surgery. It also is associated with low rates of dyspareunia. One arm of a Y-shaped mesh (typically permanent) is sutured to the anterior vagina just above the trigone, and the other arm is sutured to the posterior vagina from the level of the rectal reflection to the apex. The free end of the mesh is then affixed to the anterior longitudinal ligament of the sacrum just below the promontory using two sutures. Mesh complication rates with newer ultra-lightweight polypropylene meshes are lower than previously reported. One study of 120 women found no mesh exposure or complications at 1 year. Conventional laparoscopic and robot-assisted routes resulted in a shorter hospital stay (eg, 1–2 days versus 3–4 days), faster time to recovery, decreased blood loss, and less postoperative pain than laparotomy, with comparable short-term efficacy. A United Kingdom multicenter randomized equivalence trial compared open abdominal with laparoscopic sacral colpopexy. At 1 year, there were no differences in anatomic or subjective pelvic floor outcomes; however, blood loss, postoperative hemoglobin values, and length of hospital stay were better among the women who received laparoscopic sacral colpopexy. Based on this patient's activity level and goals, laparoscopic sacrocolpopexy would provide the best route of repair for her.

A vaginal uterosacral ligament suspension is a reasonable alternative for women with primary prolapse who are having concomitant vaginal surgery, who have risk factors for mesh-related complications (eg, smoking, immunosuppression), who place a high priority on a short recovery period, or who wish to avoid an abdominal incision. A uterosacral ligament suspension suspends the vaginal apex to the uterosacral ligaments using two to three sutures through each ligament. There are no prospective comparative studies on sacrocolpopexy and uterosacral ligament suspension; however, a recent randomized trial demonstrated similar efficacy between uterosacral ligament suspension and sacrospinous ligament suspension. The primary outcome was a composite measure of success defined as the absence of the following four factors: 1) vaginal apical descent to more than one third of the vaginal length, 2) anterior or posterior vaginal wall descent beyond the hymen, 3) bothersome vaginal bulge symptoms, and 4) retreatment of prolapse. At 2-year follow-up, there was no difference in primary outcome between uterosacral ligament and sacrospinous ligament suspension groups (surgical success 59% versus 61%; odds ratio, 0.9; 95% confidence interval, 0.6–1.5). Risks and benefits of the procedures differed slightly, with persistent neurologic pain observed more often after sacrospinous ligament suspension and ureteral obstruction more often after uterosacral ligament suspension.

Colpocleisis is a procedure that obliterates the vaginal canal in women with advanced prolapse who do not desire future vaginal intercourse. Colpocleisis is highly effective, with success rates in the range of 90–100% and decreased operative and recovery times. Given that the described patient is young and sexually active, colpocleisis would not be the best choice for her.

Iliococcygeus suspension is similar to sacrospinous ligament suspension but uses the iliococcygeus fascia over the levator plate instead of the sacrospinous ligament. Posited advantages of the iliococcygeus suspension compared with sacrospinous ligament suspension are lower risks of anterior vaginal wall recurrence and injury to the pudendal neurovascular bundle, but these benefits remain unproved. Few data are available in regard to iliococcygeus suspension. In a case–control study of 128 women with a 1–2-year follow-up, subjective success rates were similar for iliococcygeus suspension and sacrospinous ligament suspension (91% versus 94%). Objective success occurred significantly more frequently in women who underwent sacrospinous ligament suspension rather than iliococcygeus suspension (67% versus 53%).

Barber MD, Brubaker L, Burgio KL, Richter HE, Nygaard I, Weidner AC, et al. Comparison of 2 transvaginal surgical approaches and perioperative behavioral therapy for apical vaginal prolapse: the OPTIMAL randomized trial. Eunice Kennedy Shriver National Institute of Child Health and Human Development Pelvic Floor Disorders Network [published erratum appears in JAMA 2015;313:2287]. JAMA 2014;311:1023–34.

DeLancey JO, Morley GW. Total colpocleisis for vaginal eversion. Am J Obstet Gynecol 1997;176:1228–32; discussion 1232–5.

Diwadkar GB, Barber MD, Feiner B, Maher C, Jelovsek JE. Complication and reoperation rates after apical vaginal prolapse surgical repair: a systematic review [published erratum appears in Obstet Gynecol 2009;113:1377]. Obstet Gynecol 2009;113:367–73.

FitzGerald MP, Richter HE, Siddique S, Thompson P, Zyczynski H, Weber A. Colpocleisis: a review. Pelvic Floor Disorders Network. Int Urogynecol J Pelvic Floor Dysfunct 2006;17:261–71.

Freeman RM, Pantazis K, Thomson A, Frappell J, Bombieri L, Moran P, et al. A randomised controlled trial of abdominal versus laparoscopic sacrocolpopexy for the treatment of post-hysterectomy vaginal vault prolapse: LAS study. Int Urogynecol J 2013;24:377–84.

Geller EJ, Siddiqui NY, Wu JM, Visco AG. Short-term outcomes of robotic sacrocolpopexy compared with abdominal sacrocolpopexy. Obstet Gynecol 2008;112:1201–6.

Handa VL, Zyczynski HM, Brubaker L, Nygaard I, Janz NK, Richter HE, et al. Sexual function before and after sacrocolpopexy for pelvic organ prolapse. Pelvic Floor Disorders Network. Am J Obstet Gynecol 2007;197:629.e1–6.

Hsu Y, Chen L, Summers A, Ashton-Miller JA, DeLancey JO. Anterior vaginal wall length and degree of anterior compartment prolapse seen on dynamic MRI [published erratum appeared in Int Urogynecol J Pelvic Floor Dysfunct 2014;25:1447]. Int Urogynecol J Pelvic Floor Dysfunct 2008;19:137–42.

Jeon MJ, Chung SM, Jung HJ, Kim SK, Bai SW. Risk factors for the recurrence of pelvic organ prolapse. Gynecol Obstet Invest 2008;66:268–73.

Maher C, Feiner B, Baessler K, Schmid C. Surgical management of pelvic organ prolapse in women. Cochrane Database of Systematic Reviews 2013, Issue 4. Art. No.: CD004014. DOI: 10.1002/14651858. CD004014.pub5.

Maher CF, Murray CJ, Carey MP, Dwyer PL, Ugoni AM. Iliococcygeus or sacrospinous fixation for vaginal vault prolapse. Obstet Gynecol 2001;98:40–4.

Paraiso MF, Walters MD, Rackley RR, Melek S, Hugney C. Laparoscopic and abdominal sacral colpopexies: a comparative cohort study. Am J Obstet Gynecol 2005;192:1752–8.

Rooney K, Kenton K, Mueller ER, FitzGerald MP, Brubaker L. Advanced anterior vaginal wall prolapse is highly correlated with apical prolapse. Am J Obstet Gynecol 2006;195:1837–40.

Salamon CG, Lewis C, Priestley J, Gurshumov E, Culligan PJ. Prospective study of an ultra-lightweight polypropylene Y mesh for robotic sacrocolpopexy. Int Urogynecol J 2013;24:1371–5.

Summers A, Winkel LA, Hussain HK, DeLancey JO. The relationship between anterior and apical compartment support. Am J Obstet Gynecol 2006;194:1438–43.

Whiteside JL, Weber AM, Meyn LA, Walters MD. Risk factors for prolapse recurrence after vaginal repair. Am J Obstet Gynecol 2004;191:1533–8.

29

Pelvic mesh materials

Pelvic organ prolapse repair sometimes is augmented with an implantable reconstructive material to improve the durability of the reconstruction. The characteristic of the pelvic mesh that results in the lowest rate of mesh extrusion is

      (A) microporous (less than 10 microns)
      (B) high density
      (C) low elasticity
*   (D) monofilament
      (E) nonabsorbable

The use of mesh in pelvic reconstructive surgery has been the subject of considerable controversy. Of the more than 200,000 operations performed annually for pelvic organ prolapse, almost one third will require reoperation. The most durable procedure to date, abdominal sacrocolpopexy, employs mesh placed along the anterior and posterior vaginal walls and the vaginal apex and attached to the anterior longitudinal ligament on the sacrum to augment the repair. The long-term success rates of this procedure range from approximately 88% to 95%. Long-term complications are relatively uncommon; however, mesh reaction (erosion into adjacent viscera or extrusion through the vaginal tissue) can occur. The rate of this complication is related to the specific mesh material used and has decreased substantially over the past several decades as newer meshes have been introduced.

Mesh materials are classified into four types, according to weave, weight, and pore size. Most commercially available meshes today are type I, and this type of mesh has been associated with the lowest long-term erosion rates and the lowest rates of extrusion. Type I meshes are monofilament (polypropylene) in nature and are macroporous (pore size greater than 75 microns). Macropores are large enough to allow for host incorporation into the mesh with collagen deposition and angiogenesis.

Type II materials are microporous, with pore size less than 10 microns. These materials include expanded polytetrafluoroethylene and are associated with an increased extrusion rate, thought to result from the inability of fibroblasts and immune cells to penetrate the pores,

allowing collagen and connective tissue deposition only on the surface of the mesh. Microporous materials are postulated to have a higher infection risk because the small pore size limits the infiltration of large immune cells, such as macrophages.

Mesh pore size is also a determinant of material weight and elasticity. The larger the pore size, the smaller the weight and the more elastic the material. Materials with higher elasticity are thought to produce a smaller, more elastic scar. Some empiric evidence indicates that lower-weight meshes are associated with lower infection and erosion rates.

Type III multifilament meshes, such as polyethylene, are rarely used because of the increased rates of infection and erosion. Two products made with type III mesh have been removed from the market because of their unacceptably high complication rate; both products were midurethral slings used for the treatment of stress incontinence.

Absorbable materials are less likely to become infected and have less potential to harm adjacent viscera. Although use of absorbable materials, such as polyglactin or polyglycolic acid, has been attempted, animal studies show that the resultant scar tissue weakens after the material is absorbed and does not provide the long-term repair strength of a nonabsorbable material.

Amid PK. Classification of biomaterials and their related complications in abdominal wall hernia surgery. Hernia 1997;1:15–21.

Culligan PJ, Blackwell L, Goldsmith LJ, Graham CA, Rogers A, Heit MH. A randomized controlled trial comparing fascia lata and synthetic mesh for sacral colpopexy. Obstet Gynecol 2005;106:29–37.

Cundiff GW, Varner E, Visco AG, Zyczynski HM, Nager CW, Norton PA, et al. Risk factors for mesh/suture erosion following sacral colpopexy. Pelvic Floor Disorders Network. Am J Obstet Gynecol 2008;199:688.e1–5.

Iglesia CB, Fenner DE, Brubaker L. The use of mesh in gynecologic surgery. Int Urogynecol J Pelvic Floor Dysfunct 1997;8:105–15.

Trabuco EC, Klingele CJ, Gebhart JB. Xenograft use in reconstructive pelvic surgery: a review of the literature. Int Urogynecol J Pelvic Floor Dysfunct 2007;18:555–63.

30

Bowel complications after robotic sacrocolpopexy

A patient who underwent robotic sacrocolpopexy 4 days ago has nausea, vomiting, and cramping abdominal pain. On examination, she appears ill and has a tender, distended abdomen. The most appropriate initial management strategy is

      (A) exploratory laparotomy
      (B) abdominal flat plate
*   (C) computed tomography (CT) scan with contrast
      (D) diagnostic laparoscopy

Minimally invasive techniques of hysterectomy and sacrocolpopexy typically are associated with shorter recovery times; however, the gynecologic surgeon requires a high index of suspicion for intra-abdominal injury in women who deviate from a routine postoperative course of treatment. Although bowel injury is uncommon after sacrocolpopexy, early and aggressive evaluation and management can identify visceral complications after such minimally invasive surgery. Patients should not be dismissed as having a simple problem such as a gastrointestinal virus, constipation, gas pain, or narcotic sensitivity until a careful evaluation for visceral injury has been completed.

The differential diagnosis for nausea, vomiting, and abdominal pain after laparoscopic or robotic surgery includes bowel injury secondary to unrecognized enterotomy or thermal injury, small-bowel obstruction secondary to port site herniation or adhesion or else incarceration behind sacral mesh, urinoma, hematoma, and pelvic abscess. A pelvic abscess could develop as a consequence of unrecognized rectal injury during dissection of the rectovaginal space. Minimally invasive routes of surgery carry the unique risks of complications associated with blind entry into the abdominal cavity, use of thermal energy sources, and laparoscopic port insertion. In the event of an ileus after minimally invasive surgery, typically some fluid is observed in the abdominal cavity: blood, urine, or pus that is causing the resultant small-bowel distention. Awareness of this possible situation will prompt the astute gynecologic surgeon to aggressively investigate the underlying cause of a postoperative ileus.

Establishment of an accurate diagnosis will direct the appropriate subsequent medical decision making. An abdominal flat plate will serve only to demonstrate dilated loops of bowel and will not determine the underlying cause. Demonstration of free air in the abdomen on a flat plate will not confirm or refute bowel injury on postoperative day 4 because residual carbon dioxide gas from the initial surgery often is present.

The radiologic test that will most accurately determine the integrity of the genitourinary tract and gastrointestinal tract is a CT scan with intravenous and oral contrast, and this is the most appropriate test for the described patient. A CT scan without contrast is of little diagnostic benefit. If there is a high index of suspicion for bowel injury, diatrizoic acid is the preferred oral contrast media. A CT scan with intravenous and oral contrast will provide specific information about the transition point for a small-bowel obstruction such as port site herniation, whether the ureters and bladder are intact, and if a hematoma or abscess is present.

Although a patient with an acute postoperative abdomen may well require exploratory surgery, either by laparotomy or laparoscopy, a preoperative diagnosis rendered based on the appropriate imaging study will direct the most appropriate surgical care. The particular skill set of the surgical team will then direct the subsequent surgical approach by either laparoscopy or laparotomy. If imaging studies do not identify a clear source of injury and the patient remains clinically ill, however, operative intervention may be required to determine the etiology.

Barboglio PG, Toler AJ, Triaca V. Robotic sacrocolpopexy for the management of pelvic organ prolapse: a review of midterm surgical and quality of life outcomes. Female Pelvic Med Reconstr Surg 2014;20:38–43.

Shen CC, Wu MP, Lu CH, Hung YC, Lin H, Huang EY, et al. Small intestine injury in laparoscopic-assisted vaginal hysterectomy. J Am Assoc Gynecol Laparosc 2003;10:350–5.

31

Sacrospinous ligament suspension complications

A 73-year-old woman has had a vaginal bulge for 6 months. She has not experienced urinary incontinence or retention, and she reports no bowel concerns. She has diabetes mellitus and hypertension controlled with medications. She has had reconstructive pelvic surgery, including uterosacral ligament suspension. At the same time, she received a total vaginal hysterectomy and bilateral salpingo-oophorectomy. She has tried a pessary but is unable to retain one because of poor levator tone and a wide genital hiatus. On examination, her pelvic organ prolapse quantification test result is as follows:

–2	+3	+5
5	2	8
+1	+1	

She desires surgical correction and chooses to undergo a sacrospinous ligament suspension. During the procedure, after placement of two permanent sutures one fingerbreadth medial to the ischial spine along the sacrospinous ligament, brisk bleeding is encountered. The bleeding is controlled with application of topical thrombin and prolonged application of manual pressure. The sutures are then affixed to the vaginal mucosa in the standard fashion to complete the apical repair. A posterior colporrhaphy and perineorrhaphy then are performed with excellent reduction of the prolapse. In the recovery room, the patient immediately complains of severe right-sided buttock pain that radiates down the back of her leg. The best next step in management is

    (A) observation
    (B) evacuation of suspected hematoma
*   (C) release of sacrospinous sutures
    (D) proctoscopy with removal of posterior repair and perineorrhaphy sutures

Sacrospinous ligament suspension is a vaginal approach to correct vaginal vault (apical) prolapse. The procedure typically is performed unilaterally. The vaginal vault usually is attached to the right sacrospinous ligament with sutures in order to avoid the rectum on the patient's left.

The sacrospinous ligament connects the distal sacrum and coccyx to the ischial spines. The coccygeus muscle lies anterior to the sacrospinous ligament. The pudendal neurovascular bundle passes behind the ischial spine and under the lateral aspect of the sacrospinous ligament. The pudendal nerve and sacral nerve branches run parallel to the sacrospinous ligament along the ligament's superior border. The inferior gluteal artery is located

2–3 cm medial to the ischial spine (Fig. 31-1). The surgeon places two to three sutures along the distal sacrospinous ligament two fingerbreadths medial to the ischial spine in order to avoid the pudendal artery, gluteal artery, and sciatic nerves. These sutures then are passed through the fibromuscular tissue of the vagina to draw the vaginal apex toward the sacrospinous ligament.

Complications of sacrospinous ligament suspension include pain from nerve entrapment and hemorrhage, hematoma, or both. The patient's pain from nerve entrapment is likely secondary to injury of branches of the sciatic nerve. Nerve entrapment classically presents with the following triad: paresthesia, pain, and improvement with

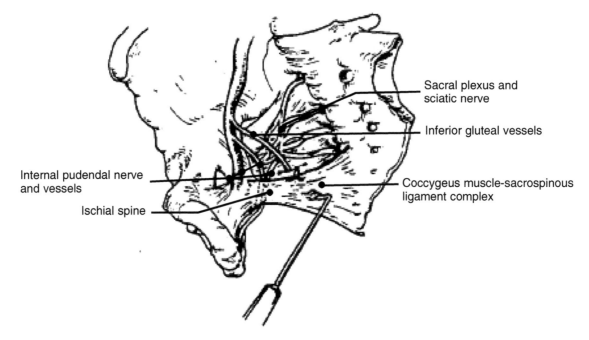

FIG. 31-1. Oblique view of the right pelvic side wall. (Miyazaki FS. Miya Hook ligature carrier for sacrospinous ligament suspension. Obstet Gynecol 1987;70:286–8.)

local anesthesia. There are ways to minimize sciatic nerve entrapment, including placing the sacrospinous sutures in a vertical rather than horizontal direction. Additionally, because the nerves travel along the superior sacrospinous ligament, the sutures should be placed in the lateral distal third of the sacrospinous ligament. Hemorrhage can be due to laceration of the interior gluteal or pudendal vessels. Such bleeding may be controlled intraoperatively with topical hemostatic agents, pressure, packing, or embolization of the bleeding vessel.

The described patient had immediate severe right-sided buttock pain in the recovery room. Observation is not recommended because to delay surgical treatment can prolong nerve entrapment and lead to permanent neuropathy. To use regional anesthesia or increase postoperative narcotics could mask the pain and delay

return to the operating room. Therefore, neither regional anesthesia nor an increase of postoperative narcotics is recommended. A hematoma is not suspected. Removal of the posterior repair and perineorrhaphy sutures will not improve the patient's pain. Return to the operating room for release of the sacrospinous sutures is the best next management step.

Barksdale PA, Elkins TE, Sanders CK, Jaramillo FE, Gasser RF. An anatomic approach to pelvic hemorrhage during sacrospinous ligament fixation of the vaginal vault. Obstet Gynecol 1998;91:715–8.

Beer M, Kuhn A. Surgical techniques for vault prolapse: a review of the literature. Eur J Obstet Gynecol Reprod Biol 2005;119:144–55.

Miyazaki FS. Miya Hook ligature carrier for sacrospinous ligament suspension. Obstet Gynecol 1987;70:286–8.

Pelvic organ prolapse. ACOG Practice Bulletin No. 85. American College of Obstetricians and Gynecologists. Obstet Gynecol 2007; 110:717–29.

32

Ectopic ureter

A 13-year-old adolescent girl is brought to your office by her mother with reports of urinary incontinence. She experiences continuous leakage of a small amount of urine during the day and overnight. She otherwise voids normally several times a day and does not have urinary urgency, frequency, or dysuria. Renal ultrasonography demonstrates a duplicated left collecting system and vaginoscopy shows a left ureteric opening into the vaginal vault. The embryonic structure that is the result of this abnormal development is the

* (A) mesonephric duct
   (B) metanephric blastema
   (C) paramesonephric duct
   (D) urogenital sinus
   (E) pronephros

Females generally have an ectopic ureter that is located distal to the striated urethral sphincter. Ectopic ureter presents in childhood (following successful bladder and bowel control) with persistent spotting or leakage of urine. Therefore, a report of continuous urinary incontinence in a girl should always elicit suspicion for a possible ectopic ureter. Ectopic ureters are more common in females than in males and are associated with a duplicated renal system in 80% of occurrences. Figure 32-1 (see color plate) illustrates common sites for an ectopic ureter in females. By contrast, males with an ectopic ureter frequently have a finding of hydronephrosis on ultrasonography or experience recurrent urinary tract infections as an infant. As a rule, males do not have urinary incontinence because the ectopic ureter is located superior to the external urinary sphincter.

Embryonically, the urinary system develops in three stages: 1) pronephros, 2) mesonephros, and 3) metanephros (Fig. 32-2; see color plate). The pronephros develops at the beginning of the fourth week of gestation and forms vestigial excretory units (ie, nephrotomes that quickly regress). At 4–5 weeks of gestation, the mesonephros develops from intermediate mesoderm. The mesonephros forms the renal corpuscle and early excretory tubules that laterally enter the longitudinal collecting mesonephric or wolffian duct and ultimately attach to the cloaca. The ureteric bud develops as an outpouching of the mesonephric duct near the cloaca. The bud penetrates newly developed metanephric tissue and dilates to form the primitive renal pelvis. The lower portion of the nephric bud migrates caudally down the mesonephric duct to connect to the bladder to form the ureters. The bladder itself develops from the anterior division of the cloaca, the urogenital sinus. Duplication of the ureter occurs when the ureteric bud splits and the induced metanephric tissue may be divided. An ectopic ureter occurs when one bud is in the normal position and the abnormal bud (associated with the more cranial renal segment) moves caudally with the mesonephric duct to form an abnormal entrance into the bladder, urethra, vestibule, or uterus. The general location of the ureteral orifice is dictated by the Weigert–Meyer rule, which acknowledges that an ectopic ureteric bud arising from an upper renal pole inserts medial and inferior to the lower pole moiety, or "upper pole, lower hole" (Fig. 32-3; see color plate). In the female, the paramesonephric duct, or müllerian duct, arises from an invagination of the urogenital ridge, running alongside the mesonephric duct (until it eventually regresses) and ultimately forming the uterus, cervix, and upper vagina.

Choudhury SR, Chadha R, Bagga D, Puri A, Debnath PR. Spectrum of ectopic ureters in children. Pediatr Surg Int 2008;24:819–23.

Keating MA. Ureteral duplication anomalies: Ectopic ureters and ureteroceles. In: Docimo SG, Canning DA, Khoury AE, editors. The Kelalis–King–Belman textbook of clinical pediatric urology. 5th ed. Boca Raton (FL): Informa Healthcare; 2007. p. 593–648.

Park JM. Normal development of the genitourinary tract. In: Wein AJ, Kavoussi LR, Novick AC, Partin AW, Peters CA, editors. Campbell-Walsh urology. 10th ed. Philadelphia (PA): Elsevier Saunders; 2012. p. 2975–3001.

Sadler TW. Urogenital system. In: Langman's medical embryology. 13th ed. Philadelphia (PA): Wolters Kluwer Health; 2015. p. 250–77.

33

Vaginal agenesis

A 17-year-old girl comes to your office with primary amenorrhea. She reports breast development at age 12 years and no cyclic pelvic pain. On examination, she has Tanner stage 4 breasts. Her external genitalia appear normal with the exception of a vaginal dimple. Ultrasonography fails to visualize a uterus. The initial laboratory test to confirm her diagnosis is her level of

  (A) follicle-stimulating hormone (FSH)
  (B) luteinizing hormone (LH)
  (C) prolactin
* (D) testosterone
  (E) dehydroepiandrosterone sulfate

Primary amenorrhea is defined as no menses by age 15 years in the setting of normal female growth patterns and normal development of secondary sex characteristics. The etiology of primary amenorrhea includes chromosomal abnormalities, hypothalamic and pituitary disease, müllerian agenesis, transverse vaginal septum or imperforate hymen, androgen insensitivity, congenital adrenal hyperplasia, and polycystic ovary syndrome.

In the described patient, who has developmental absence of the vagina and uterus and the presence of other secondary sex characteristics, the most likely diagnosis is vaginal agenesis, also referred to as müllerian agenesis, Mayer–Rokitansky–Küster–Hauser syndrome, or androgen insensitivity syndrome. Serum testosterone levels within the normal range for females can help differentiate vaginal agenesis from androgen abnormalities in which levels are elevated.

Vaginal agenesis is the result of agenesis or hypoplasia of the müllerian duct system leading to the congenital absence of the vagina and an absent or rudimentary uterus. Patients with vaginal agenesis have a normal XX karyotype and normal ovaries and, therefore, develop normal secondary sex characteristics. The external genitalia appear normal with exception of a vaginal dimple or blind vaginal pouch. Most patients present with primary amenorrhea; however, 2–7% can have an obstructed uterus with a functioning endometrium often accompanied by cyclic pelvic pain. Women with Mayer–Rokitansky–Küster–Hauser syndrome also should be evaluated for renal and skeletal anomalies, which affect 25–50% and 10–15% of patients, respectively.

Patients with androgen insensitivity syndrome have karyotype 46,XY. They have functional testes (located in the labia or inguinal area) that produce testosterone and müllerian-inhibiting substance. However, a defect in the androgen receptor leads to development of female-appearing external genitalia (generally with scant pubic hair) and breasts. Additionally, regression of müllerian structures leads to absence of a uterus, fallopian tubes, and upper vagina. Androgen insensitivity syndrome is associated with a 2–5% risk of developing testicular cancer and, therefore, patients should undergo bilateral gonadectomy after completion of puberty.

Treatment of patients with vaginal agenesis and androgen insensitivity syndrome who lack a functional vagina often involves the age-appropriate creation of a neovagina with either the use of sequentially sized vaginal dilators or surgery. Two of the most commonly performed surgeries are the McIndoe and Vecchietti procedures.

The McIndoe procedure involves harvesting a split-thickness skin graft from the thigh or buttock or the use of cadaveric tissue or dermal matrix that is then molded around a malleable stent. This is placed in a dissected perineal cavity and secured to form the vaginal orifice. Postoperatively, the stent is left in place for approximately 1 week. Surgical success is dependent on regular vaginal dilation. With appropriate postoperative care, functional success rates reach 90%.

The Vecchietti procedure may be performed abdominally through a Pfannenstiel incision or laparoscopically. The procedure involves the placement of an acrylic sphere against the vaginal dimple that is then attached to a traction device on the external abdomen by heavy gage suture material that has been tunneled through the subperitoneum. Continuous traction is placed until an appropriate caliber vagina is formed. This procedure also requires regular postoperative dilation and is associated with functional success rates as high as 98%.

Follicle-stimulating hormone and LH levels can help distinguish the etiology of amenorrhea in the setting of normal uterine anatomy. Hypothalamic dysfunction, including functional hypothalamic amenorrhea and congenital gonadotropin-releasing hormone deficiency, results in abnormal secretion of gonadotropin-releasing hormone, leading to low LH and FSH levels. By contrast, women with gonadal dysgenesis or Turner syndrome have significantly elevated FSH levels due to lack of negative feedback from ovarian secreted estradiol. Women with gonadal dysgenesis usually have normal development of the uterus and fallopian tubes but lack development of secondary sex characteristics. Serum prolactin level would be useful in diagnosing a prolactin-secreting pituitary adenoma or cranial tumor causing pituitary stalk compression. Hyperprolactinemia usually is associated with galactorrhea and most often occurs in the setting of normal pelvic anatomy. Elevated dehydroepiandrosterone sulfate levels are increased in the most common form of congenital adrenal hyperplasia, 21-hydroxylase deficiency, as well as with androgen-secreting adrenal carcinoma. For the described patient, the initial laboratory test that would confirm her diagnosis of primary amenorrhea is her level of testosterone.

Baggish MS, Karram MM. Congenital vaginal abnormalities. Congenital vaginal abnormalities. In: Atlas of pelvic anatomy and gynecologic surgery. 3rd ed. Philadelphia (PA): Elsevier Saunders; 2011. p. 811–28.

Borruto F, Camoglio FS, Zampieri N, Fedele L. The laparoscopic Vecchietti technique for vaginal agenesis. Int J Gynaecol Obstet 2007; 98:15–9.

Fritz MA, Speroff L. Amenorrhea. In: Clinical gynecologic endocrinology and infertility. 8th ed. Philadelphia (PA): Lippincott Williams & Wilkins; 2011. p. 435–94.

Klingele CJ, Gebhart JB, Croak AJ, DiMarco CS, Lesnick TG, Lee RA. McIndoe procedure for vaginal agenesis: long-term outcome and effect on quality of life. Am J Obstet Gynecol 2003;189:1569–72; discussion 1572–3.

Reindollar RH, Byrd JR, McDonough PG. Delayed sexual development: a study of 252 patients. Am J Obstet Gynecol 1981;140:371–80.

Sadler TW. Urogenital system. In: Langman's medical embryology. 13th ed. Philadelphia (PA): Wolters Kluwer Health; 2015. p. 250–77.

34

Spinal cord lesion

A 35-year-old woman with a history of spinal cord injury undergoes a cystoscopy as part of her workup for recurrent urinary tract infections. On filling the bladder to approximately 400 mL, she suddenly develops a headache and sweating on her face. Her blood pressure is 180/100 mm Hg and her heart rate is 45 beats per minute. The bladder is emptied, the cystoscope is removed, and symptoms immediately resolve. The patient likely has a spinal cord lesion located at

 * (A) cord level T4
   (B) cord level T8
   (C) spinal column level T6
   (D) spinal column level T8

People who sustain spinal cord lesions above spinal column level T6 are at risk of autonomic hyperreflexia. Such lesions arise after resolution of the spinal shock phase of a spinal cord injury and occur only in patients with a viable distal spinal cord. Autonomic hyperreflexia is an exaggerated sympathetic nervous system discharge in response to stimuli below the level of the spinal cord lesion. Such stimuli include bladder filling at the time of urodynamic testing or cystoscopy, an obstructed urinary catheter, bowel distention, or other gastrointestinal pathology. The stimulus can be pressure from tight clothing or a blood pressure cuff. Autonomic hyperreflexia occurs with headache, hypertension, flushing and sweating of the face and body above the lesion, and bradycardia. This is an emergency situation that must be dealt with immediately.

The first-line treatment is to find and reverse the precipitating stimulus, such as emptying the bladder and removing the instruments. Acute treatment of the hypertension can include alpha-adrenergic blockade, hydralazine, or nitrates.

If a patient has a known history of autonomic hyperreflexia, prophylaxis can be given before and during the necessary procedures. Procedures should be done under anesthesia with careful monitoring. Oral nifedipine can be given during and before the procedure. Chronic alpha blockade also can be used for patients who have a tendency to experience autonomic hyperreflexia.

It is important to note that the spinal cord level is not the same as the spinal column (bony spine) level (Fig. 34-1; see color plate). Spinal cord level T7–T8 corresponds to spinal column level T6. The sacral spinal cord level begins at spinal column level T12–L1, and the cauda equina begins at spinal column level L2. Because this patient has autonomic hyperreflexia, her cord lesion is above T6 cord level.

Ginsberg DA. Management of the neurogenic bladder in the female patient. Curr Urol Rep 2006;7:423–8.

Wein AJ, Demochowski RR. Neuromuscular dysfunction of the lower urinary tract. In: Wein AJ, Kavoussi LR, Novick AC, Partin AW, Peters CA, editors. Campbell-Walsh urology. 10th ed. Philadelphia (PA): Elsevier Saunders; 2012. p. 1909–46.

35

Urethral diverticula

A 48-year-old woman, para 1, with a symptomatic 5-cm urethral diverticulum requests surgical management. She also reports bothersome stress urinary incontinence. Office cystometry demonstrates urinary leakage with cough and Valsalva, 200 mL bladder volume, and maximum urethral closure pressure of 18 cm H_2O. The best concomitant anti-incontinence procedure for this patient is

    (A) periurethral bulking injection
    (B) retropubic midurethral sling
    (C) transobturator midurethral sling
    (D) laparoscopic Burch urethropexy
*   (E) autologous fascial sling

Urethral diverticula are outpouchings of the urethral mucosa. They are thought to arise from acquired defects after trauma, recurrent urinary tract infection, or surgery. They are most common in parous women and African American women. They typically present as a fluctuant anterior vaginal wall mass in a patient with dyspareunia, dysuria, postvoid dribbling, or urethral discharge. Some diverticula are asymptomatic and can be managed conservatively. Surgical repair of symptomatic urethral diverticula involves a multilayer closure with or without an interposition flap to avoid urethral stricture or urethrovaginal fistula formation. In a patient with known stress urinary incontinence, an autologous sling can serve as an additional tissue layer between the repaired urethral defect and the vaginal epithelium, thus decreasing the risk of fistula formation. In the described patient, the native tissue autologous fascial sling would be the best anti-incontinence procedure for her (Fig. 35-1; see color plate). Autologous slings are prepared using the patient's fascial tissue. Traditionally, the rectus fascia and tensor fascia lata have been used to fashion the slings.

Placement of foreign body materials should be avoided in patients with urethral diverticula because such foreign bodies increase the risk of fistula formation. For this reason, neither periurethral bulking or a synthetic midurethral sling would be acceptable procedures for this patient. Some evidence suggests that for a patient with stress incontinence (without diverticula), a retropubic

midurethral sling would be more effective than a transobturator sling in a patient with maximum urethral closure pressure less than 20 cm H_2O. A recent multicenter randomized trial comparing transobturator with retropubic midurethral slings found that retropubic slings had better long-term efficacy but also a higher rate of bladder perforation and urinary retention than transobturator slings. Autologous fascial slings are associated with a higher rate of postoperative urinary retention and voiding dysfunction than synthetic midurethral slings. Thus, if a patient wishes to minimize her risk of postoperative urinary retention, it is not unreasonable to offer her a midurethral sling at 8 weeks or more after the diverticulectomy. Staging these procedures avoids placing synthetic material against a fresh wound and diminishes the risk of fistula formation. Although a laparoscopic Burch procedure is not strictly contraindicated in this patient, such a procedure would not provide the added advantages of the fascial sling and, therefore, is not the best choice.

Albo ME, Litman HJ, Richter HE, Lemack GE, Sirls LT, Chai TC, et al. Treatment success of retropubic and transobturator mid urethral slings at 24 months. J Urol 2012;188:2281–7.

Ockrim JL, Allen DJ, Shah PJ, Greenwell TJ. A tertiary experience of urethral diverticulectomy: diagnosis, imaging and surgical outcomes. BJU Int 2009;103:1550–4.

Richter HE, Albo ME, Zyczynski HM, Kenton K, Norton PA, Sirls LT, et al. Retropubic versus transobturator 1 slings for stress incontinence. Urinary Incontinence Treatment Network. N Engl J Med 2010; 362:2066–76.

36

Lower limb peripheral nerve injury

A 58-year-old stress-continent woman has a body mass index (weight in kilograms divided by height in meters squared [kg/m^2]) of 22 and stage III pelvic organ prolapse. She undergoes an uncomplicated open supracervical hysterectomy, sacrocolpopexy, and Burch colposuspension. The surgery is done in the dorsal lithotomy position through a Pfannenstiel incision using a Balfour retractor and lasts 3 hours. On postoperative day 1, she falls as she is trying to get out of bed. She had decreased motor strength of her left quadriceps muscle (2/5), sensory loss over the anterior thigh, and an absent patellar reflex. Based on her symptoms, the nerve that has most likely been injured is

* (A) femoral
   (B) obturator
   (C) sciatic
   (D) common peroneal
   (E) ilioinguinal

The incidence of peripheral nerve injury at the time of gynecologic surgery ranges between 1.5% and 11.6%. Most lower limb neuropathies during urogynecologic surgery are transient and self-limited. Most patients with peripheral nerve injury experience complete symptom resolution. However, because long-term motor and sensory impairment can result in adverse quality of life, it is important for urogynecologic surgeons to understand the risks of lower limb nerve injury.

Most surgically induced lower limb neuropathies are a consequence of compression or stretching of a peripheral nerve and its vascular supply, which typically results in neuropraxia, the least severe type of nerve injury. Neuropraxia results from damage to the myelin sheath that creates a local conduction block with temporary loss of nerve function. Complete recovery will occur within hours or, in some cases, months after injury. Sometimes a more severe nerve injury occurs where the axon itself is injured. In axonotmesis, the axon undergoes wallerian degeneration; however, the connective tissue framework (perineurium, endoneurium, and epineurium) is intact, so over time the axon can regenerate. Axons regrow at a rate of approximately 1–2 mm per day. If the surgeon knows the site of the injury, he or she can estimate the recovery time. A rarer situation is transection of a pelvic nerve, disrupting the axon and connective tissue, resulting in the most severe nerve injury, neurotmesis, with a significantly worse prognosis.

Knowledge of the types of nerve injuries and the recovery times is important in order to counsel the patient and plan neurophysiologic consultation. Obtaining the electrodiagnostic findings necessary to differentiate neuropraxia from axonotmesis may take 3–4 weeks from the time of injury. Because most urogynecologic lower limb neuropathies are secondary to neuropraxia, they resolve without further investigation. However, early physical therapy is recommended. Risk factors associated with persistent neuropathy include prolonged surgical time, steep Trendelenburg position, low or high body mass index, a history of smoking within 20 days of the procedure, and self-retaining retractors. Lower limb neuropathies result from injury to branches of the lumbosacral plexus, including ilioinguinal, iliohypogastric, femoral, sciatic, lateral femoral cutaneous, genitofemoral, and obturator nerves.

The described patient's signs and symptoms are consistent with a femoral neuropathy. She is unable to get out of bed safely because of decreased strength in her quadriceps, sensory loss over the anterior thigh, and absent patellar reflex. The femoral nerve originates in the anterior rami of L2–L4 and provides motor innervation to the anterior compartment of the thigh and sensation to the anterior thigh and medial leg. The femoral nerve is at risk during abdominal procedures, especially when performed on thin patients through a Pfannenstiel or low-transverse incision. The femoral nerve runs through the psoas muscle and can be compressed by self-retaining retractor blades; therefore, short retractor blades are preferable. This patient has several risk factors for femoral nerve injury, including low body mass index, low-transverse incision, and self-retaining retractor blades. Femoral nerve injury can occur during vaginal surgery secondary to compression of the nerve under the inguinal ligament with excessive hip abduction, lateral rotation, or both, and hyperflexion of the thigh greater than 90 degrees.

The obturator nerve originates in the posterior rami of L2–L4, exits the pelvis through the obturator canal, and enters the thigh to supply the adductor muscles and skin over the medial thigh. The obturator nerve forms the inferior boundary of the obturator fossa and may be injured during placement of proximal paravaginal defect repair sutures. Patients with an obturator nerve injury are unable to adduct the thigh and report sensory loss over the medial thigh. Their patellar reflex remains intact.

The sciatic nerve originates in the anterior rami of L4–S4. It exits the pelvis through the greater sciatic foramen to enter the posterior compartment of the thigh and provides motor innervation to the hamstring muscles and sensation to the posterior thigh. The sciatic nerve is fixed at the sciatic notch and fibular head making it susceptible to stretch injury with hyperflexion of the thigh in stirrups. The sciatic nerve also can become entrapped in sutures during a sacrospinous ligament suspension, resulting in an entrapment neuropathy. Patients present with burning pain that radiates down the posterior thigh, decreased hamstring strength, and occasionally absent Achilles reflex. This necessitates immediate return to the operating room for suture removal.

The common peroneal nerve is one of the two terminal branches of the sciatic nerve. It exits the posterior thigh and wraps around the fibular head to innervate the anterior compartment of the leg and dorsum of the foot. It is particularly susceptible to compression and stretch injury secondary to its fixation at the fibular head. If the foot is not properly placed in the stirrup boot, the common peroneal nerve can be compressed between the fibular head and the boot and may be stretched if hyperextension at the knee occurs. Patients typically present with inversion, foot drop, and sensory loss over the anterior leg and dorsum of the foot.

The ilioinguinal nerve arises from the anterior roots of L1–L2 and provides sensation to the inguinal and suprapubic areas. The ilioinguinal nerve can become entrapped in a suture after low-transverse incisions or inferior laparoscopic trocar sites, resulting in the triad of burning pain, paresthesias, and relief with local anesthetic.

Bradshaw AD, Advincula AP. Postoperative neuropathy in gynecologic surgery. Obstet Gynecol Clin North Am 2010;37:451–9.

37

Fecal incontinence

A 65-year-old multiparous female comes to your office with accidental bowel leakage. She reports several loose stools per day with associated leakage. She has a history of anal sphincter laceration with her first delivery 40 years ago. The intervention that is most likely to eliminate her fecal incontinence is

  (A) overlapping anal sphincteroplasty
* (B) loperamide
  (C) sacral neuromodulation
  (D) biofeedback
  (E) posterior levatorplasty

Recent studies confirm that advancing age is the most important risk factor for accidental bowel leakage. Although the overall prevalence of fecal incontinence among noninstitutionalized men and women in the United States is approximately 9%, prevalence linearly increases with age from 2.9% among individuals aged 20–29 years to 16.2% in individuals older than 70 years. This corresponds to a sixfold increased risk in women aged 70 years or older.

In addition to advancing age, other consistent risk factors for accidental bowel leakage include loose stool or diarrhea (at least threefold increased risk), type 2 diabetes mellitus, body mass index (weight in kilograms divided by height in meters squared [kg/m^2]) greater than 30, and multiple chronic medical illnesses. Diabetes mellitus may adversely affect bowel control through neuropathic decompensation or potentially as a consequence of altered bowel motility secondary to medications (metformin hydrochloride) or bacterial overgrowth. In the case of the described patient, the presence of multiple loose stools per day suggests that the primary contributing factor to her fecal incontinence is abnormal stool consistency and motility.

Younger women may suffer from accidental bowel leakage as a consequence of obstetric trauma, yet even women who sustain a complete anal sphincter tear have only been noted to have a twofold long-term increased risk of bowel leakage. The interaction between anal sphincter injury and diarrhea may present a far greater challenge to the fecal continence mechanism than the presence of either in isolation. In a population study of women with irritable bowel syndrome, the synergistic interactions of anal sphincter tears with fecal urgency and diarrhea were found to act together to present a significant risk factor for fecal incontinence. It is certainly plausible that the "tipping point" for a woman with anal sphincter injury from continence to accidental bowel leakage is highly dependent on the consistency of stool that is delivered to the rectum. Medical control of diarrhea is paramount for symptom control in these women.

Biofeedback with or without electrical stimulation has demonstrated a positive effect on fecal incontinence. Biofeedback can improve rectal sensation and sphincter strength and endurance. The best intervention for this patient, however, is to control stool consistency and motility with the use of loperamide, an opioid receptor agonist that stimulates receptors in the myenteric plexus of the large intestine to decrease smooth muscle tone. This results in increased time for substances to stay in the intestine, allowing for more water to be absorbed out of the fecal matter. Loperamide also decreases colonic mass movements and suppresses the gastrocolic reflex. Once the patient's stool consistency is improved, biofeedback then would be recommended for continued fecal incontinence management.

Surgical management of fecal incontinence has yielded disappointing results. In long-term studies of overlapping anal sphincteroplasty, fewer than one half of the patients remained continent. This is likely a reflection of the fact that the external anal sphincter only provides 25% of the tone of the anal canal and cannot protect against loss of liquid stool and gas. Similarly, posterior levatorplasty and gracioloplasty are not associated with positive long-term outcomes. In this patient with loose stools, any type of surgical management would be inadvisable as a first-line intervention.

The advent of neuromodulation has been touted as a viable treatment option, with success rates of 80–83%, yet the higher costs of such treatment potentially limit widespread applicability. In addition, women with consistently loose stools are more likely to benefit from simple reversal of this problem with drug therapy as compared with surgical management using neuromodulation. Another minimally invasive surgical option that has received U.S. Food and Drug Administration approval for management of fecal incontinence is the injection of dextranomer in stabilized sodium hyaluronate, essentially a gel, under the anoderm to increase anal resistance. A Cochrane review reported that one large randomized trial found a short-term benefit in just over one half of the patients studied. To date, no long-term studies have been done.

Heymen S, Scarlett Y, Jones K, Ringel Y, Drossman D, Whitehead WE. Randomized controlled trial shows biofeedback to be superior to pelvic floor exercises for fecal incontinence. Dis Colon Rectum 2009;52:1730–7.

Matthews CA, Whitehead WE, Townsend MK, Grodstein F. Risk factors for urinary, fecal, or dual incontinence in the Nurses' Health Study. Obstet Gynecol 2013;122:539–45.

Omar MI, Alexander CE. Drug treatment for faecal incontinence in adults. Cochrane Database of Systematic Reviews 2013, Issue 6. Art. No.: CD002116. DOI: 10.1002/14651858.CD002116.pub2.

38

Rectovaginal fistula

A 30-year-old healthy woman visits your office with gas and loose stool per vagina 4 weeks after fourth-degree repair after a vaginal delivery. She is found to have a 7-mm rectovaginal fistula above the anal sphincter complex. The most appropriate management is

    (A) temporary diverting colostomy
    (B) expectant management for 3 months
*   (C) mobilization of fistula tract and layered closure
    (D) fibrin plug
    (E) high-fiber diet

Postpartum rectovaginal fistulas typically develop as a consequence of perineal wound breakdown or from unrecognized rectal injury sustained during an instrumental delivery. A rectal examination after each vaginal delivery is paramount to recognition of "button-hole" injuries to the rectal mucosa that develop into rectovaginal fistulas if left untreated. Up to 5% of fourth-degree perineal tears are complicated by wound breakdown. Identified risk factors include diabetes mellitus, smoking, and forceps delivery.

The passage of liquid and solid stool through the vagina can have a devastating emotional effect on a new mother. Other symptoms that are suggestive of a rectovaginal fistula include passage of gas and mucus material through the vagina and chronic vaginal discharge from bacterial contamination. Women with reports of gas via the vagina, however, may not always demonstrate a fistula. Vaginal flatus is a well-recognized entity and occurs when air enters the introitus and gets trapped inside the vaginal canal. When the air audibly evacuates, typically with movement, it may cause considerable social embarrassment. Obstetricians should consider this diagnosis if there is no evidence of a fistula on physical examination or after appropriate diagnostic testing.

Postpartum obstetric fistulas typically are evident on careful vaginal inspection as they occur in the lower one third of the vagina. A Sims speculum is useful for exposure of the posterior vaginal wall. Any areas of dimpling, scarring, stellate retraction, or granulation tissue should be investigated carefully with a lacrimal duct probe. Digital rectal examination may reveal an area where the rectal mucosa is tethered to the vagina. If a fistula tract is not visible, methylene blue dye may be instilled into the rectum using a bulb syringe to observe where it appears on the posterior vaginal wall. The size and location of the

fistula in relation to the anal sphincter complex should be noted because this may affect the repair. If the sphincter is involved, the repair should include identification and repair of the internal and external anal sphincters.

Surgical management of postpartum rectovaginal fistulas has evolved with time. Historically, surgeons recommended that women wait at least 3 months for definitive surgical repair to reduce tissue inflammation and theoretically improve the chance of surgical success. More contemporary studies, however, report good outcomes with early surgical intervention using a simple layered approach as long as no active infection is present. This is the best management for the described patient, who should receive mobilization of the fistula tract and layered closure. Pinpoint fistulas (less than 4 mm) have up to a 40% chance of spontaneous closure, so a period of expectant management is advisable in such cases. Fistulas that are larger than 5 mm in size, however, rarely close without surgical intervention.

Fibrin material placed through the fistula tract is a newer method of repair and has been used primarily in patients with inflammatory bowel disease. To date, no prospective comparative trials have been reported that compare traditional layered surgical repair with fibrin plug repair. A fibrin plug would not be the best option for the described patient. Temporary fecal diversion typically is only recommended in women with inflammatory bowel disease who have failed an initial attempt at repair.

Gajsek U, McArthur DR, Sagar PM. Long-term efficacy of the button fistula plug in the treatment of Ileal pouch-vaginal and Crohn's-related rectovaginal fistulas. Dis Colon Rectum 2011;54:999–1002.

Sjoveian S, Vangen S, Mukwege D, Onsrud M. Surgical outcome of obstetric fistula: a retrospective analysis of 595 patients. Acta Obstet Gynecol Scand 2011;90:753–60.

39

Upper limb nerve injury

A 48-year-old woman with stage III uterovaginal prolapse is scheduled for a robotic-assisted laparoscopic supracervical hysterectomy and abdominal sacrocervicopexy followed by perineorrhaphy and placement of a midurethral sling. Before the procedure, she is positioned on the table with foam padding to secure her torso, along with shoulder rests to assure that she does not slip up the table while she is in a steep Trendelenburg position. The hysterectomy is difficult because of a uterine fibroid and multiple adhesions that require an additional 30 minutes of lysis of adhesions. The entire surgical procedure lasted 6 hours. During rounds the next day, the patient tells you that she is unable to pick up her coffee cup with her right hand, although she has no pain. The best next step in management is

      (A) observation

      (B) thoracic magnetic resonance imaging

*   (C) physical therapy

      (D) neuropathic pain medication

      (E) surgical reattachment of the affected nerve

Nerve injury during urogynecologic surgery occurs with stretching or compression of the nerve, entrapment caused by suture placement, transection, or thermal injury. With advanced laparoscopic and robotic-assisted procedures, the brachial plexus is at risk of injury caused by pressure, stretching, or compression. Brachial plexus neuropathy occurs as a result of stretching of the brachial plexus if a patient slides cephalad when she is in a steep Trendelenburg position with her arms fixed to her sides. Shoulder blocks can place direct pressure on the nerves if placed too medially; therefore, the blocks should have pressure directed on the acromial processes.

Typically, the patient will have motor weakness and a sensory deficit in the distribution of the affected nerve. The described patient has signs of a brachial plexus nerve injury with weakness in unilateral upper motor functioning. This compression nerve injury was most likely caused by improper positioning or padding of the patient's shoulders in the operating room, with the prolonged surgical time resulting in ischemia. Pressure from shoulder straps or blocks can compress the brachial nerve. The typical presentation of a brachial nerve injury is painless and involves weakness of one of the upper extremities.

Most patients will experience complete recovery. The best initial approach is to have the patient undergo physical therapy. The duration of the neuropathy depends on the degree to which the nerve was affected by a hypoxic insult, but with time, the injury should resolve spontaneously without lasting damage or persistent symptoms. Thoracic magnetic resonance imaging will not provide information on the nerve function. Neuropathic pain medications are not necessary given that the described patient reports weakness but no pain. The nerve injury is from a compression injury and not a transection, so no surgical reattachment is needed.

Bradshaw AD, Advincula AP. Postoperative neuropathy in gynecologic surgery. Obstet Gynecol Clin North Am 2010;37:451–9.

Ferrante MA. Brachial plexopathies: classification, causes, and consequences. Muscle Nerve 2004;30:547–68.

40
Nocturia

An 82-year-old woman, para 4, with nighttime urinary urgency and frequency tells you that she is awakened four to five times every night with the need to go to the toilet. She experiences urinary incontinence on occasion, despite "running to the bathroom." She does not have bothersome urinary symptoms during the daytime. In addition to keeping a voiding diary, you tell her that the best next step is

     (A) oral desmopressin
*   (B) bedside commode for nighttime use
     (C) intradetrusor botulinum toxin A injection
     (D) oral oxybutynin at bedtime
     (E) percutaneous tibial nerve stimulation

Nocturia is defined as two or more episodes of being awakened during the night with an urge to void. Patients with nocturia report lower quality-of-life scores and increased symptoms of depression. Nocturia is more prevalent in the elderly and is commonly multifactorial. It can result from various causes, such as excessive fluid intake in the evening, congestive heart failure, venous insufficiency, medication adverse effects, obstructive sleep apnea, restless leg syndrome, desmopressin deficiency, or bladder outlet obstruction. Whereas in men, benign prostatic hypertrophy is a common cause of bladder outlet obstruction leading to nocturia, women with high-grade pelvic organ prolapse can experience nocturia when reduction of prolapse in the supine position facilitates bladder emptying. A voiding diary or frequency–volume diary can differentiate nocturia from nocturnal polyuria. A patient has nocturnal polyuria if more than 35% of her 24-hour urine volume is voided at night. Treatment to target the underlying causes of nocturnal polyuria can improve the patient's symptoms. A voiding diary is a useful source of diagnostic clues and helps to track response to therapy.

In older women, nocturia and nighttime urinary urgency commonly cause falls and associated fractures. It is important to counsel this patient, who reports hurrying to the bathroom at night, on fall prevention. A hip fracture in a patient of this age is associated with a 50% mortality rate within the first year after the fracture. Hip fractures are also a common cause of institutionalization in the elderly. The best way to minimize her risk of nighttime falls will be for her to use a bedside commode.

Oral desmopressin produces modest improvement of nocturia symptoms in patients with nocturnal polyuria compared with placebo treatment. Close monitoring during desmopressin therapy is necessary to identify hyponatremia, a potentially life-threatening complication of treatment. Because of these complications, desmopressin treatment is reserved for patients with idiopathic or refractory nocturia and would not be the appropriate next step for this patient.

Oral anticholinergics are rarely more effective than placebo in reducing nocturia. Additionally, adverse effects, including confusion and poor balance, are not uncommon with anticholinergics. For this patient to take oral oxybutynin at bedtime may place her at even higher risk of falls. Percutaneous tibial nerve stimulation, oxybutynin, and botulinum toxin A injection are effective treatments for overactive bladder. Although this patient has nighttime urinary urgency, she denies overactive bladder symptoms during the daytime, so none of these types of therapy are appropriate for her.

Ebell MH, Radke T, Gardner J. A systematic review of the efficacy and safety of desmopressin for nocturia in adults. J Urol 2014;192:829–35.

Weiss JP, Blaivas JG, Blanker MH, Bliwise DL, Dmochowski RR, Drake M, et al. The New England Research Institutes, Inc. (NERI) Nocturia Advisory Conference 2012: focus on outcomes of therapy. BJU Int 2013;111:700–16.

41

Rectal prolapse

An 80-year-old woman who underwent colpocleisis 1 year ago comes to your office with intermittent fecal incontinence. She reports a sensation of incomplete bowel evacuation and rectal fullness. The most likely finding on physical examination is

   (A) prolapsing internal hemorrhoids
 * (B) rectal prolapse
   (C) posterior wall prolapse
   (D) rectal intussusception

In elderly patients who no longer desire sexual function, obliterative surgery for pelvic organ prolapse is associated with reduced operative morbidity and higher anatomic cure rates than reconstructive surgery. Most studies report success rates of 90–100%. Recurrent vaginal prolapse of any compartment is uncommon. Therefore, this patient is unlikely to have either a rectocele or enterocele on her examination at 1 year postsurgery.

Rectal prolapse is defined as a full-thickness protrusion of the rectum through the anus. The prevalence in the general population is estimated to be less than 0.5%. A significantly higher rate, however, has been reported in women who undergo colpocleisis compared with reconstructive vaginal procedures. A reasonable proposed theory to explain the observed association is that narrowing of the genital hiatus and obliteration of the vagina results in displacement of intra-abdominal pressure through the remaining pelvic opening, the anus. With the vaginal canal blocked off, pelvic viscera then are displaced through the remaining "path of least resistance," and rectal prolapse results. It also is possible that elderly women who are selected for an obliterative as opposed to reconstructive surgical procedure represent a higher-risk population with inherently weak and debilitated tissue and, therefore, are at risk of other forms of prolapse. Although internal hemorrhoids would be the most likely answer in a woman without a history of colpocleisis, the unique association between colpocleisis and subsequent rectal prolapse suggests that rectal prolapse is the most likely diagnosis in this case.

The clinical presentation of rectal prolapse is varied. Complete external rectal prolapse is associated with a large red or pink rectal mass or visible bulge (Fig. 41-1; see color plate). The bulge may or may not spontaneously reduce after a bowel movement. Less obvious cases, however, typically are associated with nonspecific complaints such as rectal fullness, rectal pressure, pelvic heaviness, a sensation of incomplete rectal evacuation, mucus discharge, fecal incontinence, and rectal bleeding. Many of these symptoms are very similar to those seen in women with posterior compartment prolapse of the vagina.

Rectal prolapse is a clinical diagnosis that should be suspected based on the patient's presenting symptoms and surgical history. It often is not reproducible in the lithotomy position and, thus, the patient always should be examined when straining on a commode. In the event that rectal prolapse still is not evident, defecography should be ordered to investigate for rectal intussusception and internal rectal prolapse. Additional diagnostic investigations should include a colonoscopy to rule out the presence of a lead point, such as a colonic mass or other pathology, that may change the surgical approach.

In addition to causing patient discomfort, rectal prolapse can result in bowel incarceration. Earlier repair generally is advised because chronic externalization of the rectal mucosa can result in tissue inflammation, increased bleeding and ulceration, and gradual distention and weakening of the anal sphincter, predisposing the patient to postoperative fecal incontinence.

The two major surgical approaches for the correction of rectal prolapse are 1) intra-abdominal rectopexy using suture or mesh or 2) a transperineal approach. Much like vaginal prolapse repair, the abdominal route for rectal prolapse is associated with improved outcomes but higher surgical morbidity. The two transperineal procedures, Altemeier and Delorme, typically are reserved for elderly patients with significant comorbidities. In the United States, the Altemeier procedure is performed more commonly than the Delorme procedure.

In the Altemeier technique, a full-thickness circumferential incision is made above the dentate line, the rectum is dissected until the peritoneal cavity is reached, the redundant floppy bowel is resected, and the coloanal anastomosis is sewn. In patients who have undergone colpocleisis, in which the rectum is approximated to the bladder, this procedure probably will not be feasible.

The Delorme technique involves mucosal stripping by dissection in the submucosal layer of the rectum followed by plication of the rectal muscularis and an anastomosis of the proximal mucosal layer and the anal canal proximal to the dentate line.

Bordeianou L, Hicks CW, Kaiser AM, Alavi K, Sudan R, Wise PE. Rectal prolapse: an overview of clinical features, diagnosis, and patient-specific management strategies. J Gastrointest Surg 2014;18:1059–69.

Collins SA, Jelovsek JE, Chen CC, Gustilo-Ashby AM, Barber MD. De novo rectal prolapse after obliterative and reconstructive vaginal surgery for urogenital prolapse. Am J Obstet Gynecol 2007;197:84.e1–3.

42

Urinary diversion

A 35-year-old woman had a diving accident 2 years ago, resulting in a complete T9 spinal cord injury. Immediately after the accident, she developed acute urinary retention requiring an indwelling urethral catheter. After she recovered from her injuries, she was taught clean intermittent catheterization, which she performed without any issues until 1 year after the accident, at which time she developed urinary incontinence between catheterizations. Her incontinence was controlled with anticholinergic agents for nearly 12 months. However, more recently, she has developed progressively worse leakage between catheterizations. Urodynamic tests demonstrate poor compliance, with detrusor pressure increasing to 50 cm H_2O at a volume of 150 mL and a detrusor leak point pressure of 60 cm H_2O at a volume of 200 mL. She has no leakage with cough or Valsalva maneuver. Renal ultrasonography reveals mild bilateral hydronephrosis. The best next step in management is

        (A) increase anticholinergic agents
        (B) increase rate of clean intermittent catheterization
*   (C) ileocystoplasty
        (D) augmentation cystoplasty with continent cutaneous stoma
        (E) ileal conduit urinary diversion

After a spinal cord injury, the bladder goes through a period of acute spinal shock for 6–12 weeks in which the bladder is atonic and does not empty. This often is managed in the short term with an indwelling Foley catheter while the patient recovers from other associated injuries. As soon as feasible, patients are taught clean intermittent catheterization. The process usually is performed five times a day, with the goal of keeping the bladder volume below 500 mL. If a patient drinks high volumes of fluid, more frequent catheterizations may be needed. Some patients may regain the ability to void after the spinal shock phase is over. Over time, as the cord lesion evolves, patients most frequently develop detrusor sphincter dyssynergia, in which the bladder contracts against a closed external sphincter, resulting in urinary retention, pressure on the upper urinary tract, urge urinary incontinence, and overflow incontinence from inability to empty.

The best initial management of detrusor sphincter dyssynergia is clean intermittent catheterization combined with anticholinergic agents. The catheterization empties the bladder and the anticholinergic agents decrease urge contractions, making this ideal long-term management

for the patient with detrusor sphincter dyssynergia who is able to self-catheterize. Leakage between catheterizations is the chief reason for failure of clean intermittent catheterization with anticholinergics. Leakage between catheterizations is caused by one of two conditions: 1) detrusor overactivity between catheterizations, which is often high-pressure overactivity that does not respond to anticholinergics, or 2) poor bladder compliance. Patients who leak between catheterizations because of poor bladder compliance demonstrate on urodynamic testing a slow increase in bladder pressure with filling versus intermittent overactive contractions. *Detrusor leak point pressure* is defined at the lowest value of detrusor pressure at which leakage is observed in the absence of strain or detrusor contraction. Based on studies in the pediatric population, patients whose bladder pressures increase to over 40 cm H_2O with filling up of detrusor pressure before leakage occurs (ie, those who experience a detrusor leak point pressure over 40 cm H_2O) are at risk of upper urinary tract damage. Both causes of leakage between catheterizations warrant surgical management. The described patient has high pressures at low volumes and has a high detrusor pressure at maximum flow, indicating risk to her kidneys. Increasing the rate of clean intermittent catheterization is unlikely to help her symptoms and is not practical.

Because this patient catheterizes successfully, ileocystoplasty will provide the best solution with minimal complications (Fig. 42-1). This procedure involves opening the bladder widely and patching it with a U-shaped segment of ileum in order to restore bladder capacity. If a patient has difficulty with self-catheterization by means of the urethra, augmentation cystoplasty can be performed with a catheterizable stoma (ie, a continent cutaneous bladder augmentation). However, there is a high rate of stomal complications with continent cutaneous bladder augmentations, including stomal stenosis and stomal incontinence. An ideal conduit requires bilateral ureteral reimplantation but is a good choice for patients who desire an incontinent diversion and whose urine needs to be totally diverted (ie, their native bladder cannot be used). Certain patients are at high risk of leakage through the urethra and are not reconstructable, such as in the case of a large urethral erosion from a Foley catheter. Continent diversions with a catheterizable stoma are an option for such patients (Fig. 42-2).

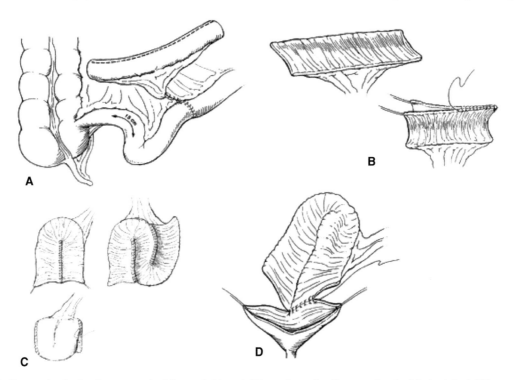

FIG. 42-1. Ileocystoplasty. A segment of ileum (at least 15 cm from the ileocecal valve) is isolated **(A)**, opened, and fashioned to create a large patch **(B** and **C)**. After opening the bladder in a "clam-shell" configuration **(D)**, the augment is sewn to the native bladder. (Abou-Elela A. Augmentation cystoplasty in pretransplant recipients. In: Ortiz J, Andre J, editors. Understanding the complexities of kidney transplantation. Rijeka, Croatia: INTECH Open Access Publisher; 2011. Available at: http://www.intechopen.com/books/understanding-the-complexities-of-kidney-transplantation/augmentation-cystoplasty-in-pretransplant-recepients. Retrieved October 7, 2015.)

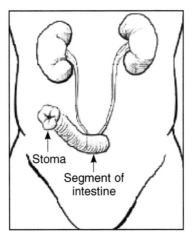

FIG. 42-2. Ileal conduit urinary diversion. (Reprinted with permission, Cleveland Clinic Center for Medical Art & Photography. Copyright 2016 All Rights Reserved.)

Dahl DM, McDougal WS. Use of intestinal segments in urinary diversion. In: Wein AJ, Kavoussi LR, Novick AC, Partin AW, Peters CA, editors. Campbell–Walsh urology. 10th ed. Philadelphia (PA): Elsevier Saunders; 2012. p. 2411–49.

Wein AJ, Demochowski RR. Neuromuscular dysfunction of the lower urinary tract. In: Wein AJ, Kavoussi LR, Novick AC, Partin AW, Peters CA, editors. Campbell-Walsh urology. 10th ed. Philadelphia (PA): Elsevier Saunders; 2012. p. 1909–46.

43

Detrusor sphincter dyssynergia

A 50-year-old woman was diagnosed with multiple sclerosis after an episode of acute urinary retention. She was initially managed with an indwelling catheter for 2 weeks, after which she was taught clean intermittent catheterization. Three months later, she regained the ability to void again and was fully continent. However, over the next 6 months she developed voiding difficulty with periodic leakage in which she totally emptied her bladder in her wheelchair. At her office visit, her postvoid residual urine volume was 400 mL. She returned to the office 1 week later for urodynamic testing. Before emptying her with a catheter, her initial postvoid residual urine volume was 450 mL. Her urodynamic testing demonstrates the tracing illustrated in Figure 43-1 (see color plate). The best next step in management for her is

      (A) augmentation cystoplasty
      (B) indwelling Foley catheter
*   (C) clean intermittent catheterization and anticholinergic agent
      (D) suprapubic tube placement

Urodynamic testing is useful in determining the etiology of the patient's voiding dysfunction. Multiple sclerosis can affect voiding and storage in a multitude of ways, depending on the exact location of the affected white matter lesions. Neurologic lesions above the pons (the micturition center of the brain), regardless of etiology, typically result in detrusor overactivity with external sphincter synergy. This results in urinary urgency incontinence, but there is no danger to the upper urinary tract. Lesions in the spinal cord cause detrusor sphincter dyssynergia, causing a combination of detrusor overactivity with impaired emptying. This can result in elevated bladder pressures and risk to the kidneys. The urodynamic tracing in Figure 43-1 (see color plate) shows classic detrusor sphincter dyssynergia. With each increase in detrusor pressure, there is an increase in external sphincter tone, as evidenced by electromyography. This results not only in urinary retention but also potential danger to the upper urinary tract from high filling pressures. Optimal initial management of detrusor sphincter dyssynergia is clean intermittent catheterization in combination with anticholinergic agent therapy. The anticholinergic agent helps to stop or reduce the frequency of detrusor contractions with filling and thereby increases bladder capacity and reduces leakage episodes. Clean intermittent catheterization will empty the bladder completely and usually is recommended five times daily so that the bladder volume does not increase significantly. Ideally, bladder volume should not exceed 500 mL, so clean intermittent catheterization can be performed more frequently, if needed, depending on the patient's fluid intake.

The described patient initially had a period of urinary retention and was able to self-catheterize successfully. Based on her urodynamic findings consistent with detrusor sphincter dyssynergia, her current neurologic lesion is located in the spinal cord. In addition, she is leaking as a result of her high-pressure bladder contractions and, possibly, overflow incontinence from not emptying. Since she was able to catheterize herself in the past without event, clean intermittent catheterization combined with anticholinergic therapy is the best next step for her.

An indwelling Foley catheter would be the best short-term step for patients who are unable to catheterize and who are waiting for definitive surgical management. Suprapubic tube placement would not provide ideal long-term management in a healthy 50-year-old woman with a long life expectancy but is less traumatic on the urethra than an indwelling Foley catheter, which can lead to urethral erosion. Augmentation cystoplasty would be an option for a patient who leaks between catheterizations, but it is not the best next step for someone who has not tried clean intermittent catheterization or anticholinergics.

Wein AJ, Demochowski RR. Neuromuscular dysfunction of the lower urinary tract. In: Wein AJ, Kavoussi LR, Novick AC, Partin AW, Peters CA, editors. Campbell-Walsh urology. 10th ed. Philadelphia (PA): Elsevier Saunders; 2012. p. 1909–46.

44

Cystoscopy

A 52-year-old woman is undergoing a midurethral retropubic synthetic sling placement for stress urinary incontinence. Immediately after trocar placement, gross hematuria is noted in the Foley catheter. With the use of a 70-degree lens, cystoscopy is performed and reveals bilateral perforations of the sling trocars. The passers then are removed. Repeat cystoscopy reveals ongoing brisk bleeding from the left-sided trocar site, resulting in red-colored urine. The best next step is

        (A) abandon the sling procedure
*   (B) replace the sling
        (C) continuous bladder irrigation for 48 hours
        (D) abdominal repair by cystotomy

The equipment needed to carry out cystoscopy includes a lens, sheath, light cord, and light source, together with a working bridge that allows for instrument passage. Sterile water or saline is attached to tubing, which then enters the bladder through the sheath and fills the bladder. Historically, the naked eye was used to visualize the bladder and urethra through the lens. Today, it is more common to use a camera that connects to a video tower for ease of viewing. Initial placement of the sheath is aided by use of an obturator, which allows smooth placement of the cystoscope. The lens, camera, and light cord are attached after the cystoscope sheath is in the bladder. The bladder is filled to capacity so that all components of the urothelium can be visualized. The exact technique of bladder inspection is based on surgeon preference. The surgeon must be sure that the entire bladder is visualized, including the bladder neck and urethra. A 0-degree or 30-degree lens will best visualize the urethra. The bladder then is inspected with a 70-degree lens. At the time of placement of the sling, cystoscopy should focus initially on the dome of the bladder. For otherwise routine cystoscopy, attention is first directed to the trigone. Both ureteral orifices are identified, and efflux of urine is seen. Then the camera is rotated slowly so that the entirety of the bladder is visualized. With each 45-degree rotation, care is taken to visualize a large segment of mucosa that extends from the posterior bladder wall all the way to the bladder neck. This will ensure that no bladder lesions are missed. This is continued for 360 degrees, until the entirety of the bladder is visualized.

Cystoscopy should be a part of every sling operation to ensure that there is no passage of trocars or sling material into the bladder. Trocar passage through the bladder happens frequently during retropubic sling surgery (incidence of approximately 5%). It is generally of no consequence, provided the injury is recognized and the trocars repassed. Missing a trocar injury can be avoided by using a 70-degree cystoscopy lens and looking carefully at the dome of the bladder (trocars will be located at the 11-o'clock and 1-o'clock positions at both sides of the dome). Inspection should occur with a full bladder, because a partially empty bladder may not allow for visualization of a trocar injury. Wiggling the abdominal side of the trocar during cystoscopy can help identify where the trocar is located relative to the bladder. Should a trocar be seen in the bladder, the surgeon should then empty the bladder and repass the trocars. Repeat cystoscopy will confirm that the repeat passage of the trocar was performed correctly and the trocar is no longer in the bladder.

Occasionally, trocar passage into the bladder can result in gross hematuria. Usually, it remits without the need for coagulation. If bladder visibility is poor, the bladder can be irrigated by carefully emptying and refilling the bladder with the cystoscope sheath. Alternatively, a syringe with a catheter mount (with an adapter) can be used to irrigate the bladder through the cystoscopy sheath (Fig. 44-1; see color plate). However, the surgeon must be careful to avoid excess irrigation, given the fact that there is a bladder perforation from which fluid can leak out of the bladder. If bleeding persists despite these maneuvers, a monopolar, flexible electrode can be placed through the cystoscope and used to coagulate the bleeding vessel at the trocar perforation site.

45

Posterior vaginal wall prolapse

A 58-year-old woman comes to your office with a vaginal bulge that she has felt for the past year. In order to defecate, she has to use her fingers to push on her perineum and inside her vagina. She tells you, "It feels like my stool is getting stuck." She has not experienced bowel leakage. She has no significant prior medical history and has never had surgery. She is sexually active. She had a forceps delivery of a 3,629-g (8-lb) infant and recalls a tear into her rectum. A rectovaginal examination demonstrates a distal pocket and laxity. She desires definitive surgical management. On examination, her pelvic organ prolapse quantification test result is as follows:

–2	–2	–7
4	2	10
+3	+4	–8

You recommend

* (A) posterior colporrhaphy
  (B) graft-augmented site-specific posterior vaginal wall repair
  (C) sacral colpoperineopexy
  (D) transanal rectocele repair

This patient has stage III posterior vaginal wall prolapse. She is symptomatic from bulge and obstructed defecation, specifically splinting, or the need to use her fingers in her vagina, perineum, or rectum to facilitate stool emptying. The goal of surgical correction is to fix the underlying anatomic defect by reducing the bulge and to correct any associated symptoms of obstructed defecation (splinting, manual evacuation, and straining).

Surgical options for distal posterior vaginal wall defects include traditional posterior colporrhaphy, site-specific defect repair, graft augmentation, and colpoperineopexy, if there is an apical component. Posterior colporrhaphy involves plicating the posterior vaginal fibromuscular layer, possibly with levator ani plication, perineorrhaphy, or both. This procedure has a success rate of 76–96%. Site-specific defect repair seeks to identify and repair specific tears in the rectovaginal septum with individual stitches and has a success rate of 82% or higher. Graft augmentation has been used in isolation or in combination with a posterior colporrhaphy or site-specific repair. Grafts have been attached proximally to apical sutures in the sacrospinous ligament, arcus tendineus, fascia rectovaginalis, or cervix. In women with an apical component to their posterior vaginal wall prolapse, a sacral colpoperineopexy, in which the posterior arm of synthetic mesh is extended down the posterior vaginal wall dissection and attached to the perineal body,

can be performed. Colorectal surgeons have approached posterior vaginal wall prolapse with a transanal approach as opposed to the vaginal approach to achieve posterior colporrhaphy.

A randomized controlled trial compared posterior colporrhaphy, site-specific defect repair, and porcine graft augmentation. One year after surgery, the cure rates of posterior colporrhaphy (86%) and site-specific repair (78%) were significantly better than those for graft augmentation (54%). Based on this study and others showing increased pain and complications with mesh, graft use is not recommended in the posterior compartment. Levator plication is not recommended in sexually active women due to high dyspareunia rates. Posterior colporrhaphy is the best procedure for the described patient with stage III posterior vaginal wall prolapse.

Maher C, Feiner B, Baessler K, Schmid C. Surgical management of pelvic organ prolapse in women. Cochrane Database of Systematic Reviews 2013, Issue 4. Art. No.: CD004014. DOI: 10.1002/14651858. CD004014.pub5.

Murphy M. Clinical practice guidelines on vaginal graft use from the society of gynecologic surgeons. Society of Gynecologic Surgeons Systematic Review Group. Obstet Gynecol 2008;112:1123–30.

Paraiso MF, Barber MD, Muir TW, Walters MD. Rectocele repair: a randomized trial of three surgical techniques including graft augmentation. Am J Obstet Gynecol 2006;195:1762–71.

Pelvic organ prolapse. ACOG Practice Bulletin No. 85. American College of Obstetricians and Gynecologists. Obstet Gynecol 2007;110:717–29.

46

Vertebral discitis

A 45-year-old woman comes to the emergency department 5 months after undergoing a robotic-assisted laparoscopic sacrocolpopexy. She reports back pain and lower extremity pain and weakness. On examination, she is afebrile with tenderness over the lumbosacral spine and normal neurologic function. Spinal magnetic resonance imaging reveals increased L5–S1 vertebral body and intervertebral disc enhancement on T2 weighted images. The most likely microbial pathogen associated with her vertebral discitis is

- (A) *Candida albicans*
- (B) group B *Streptococcus*
- (C) *Mycobacterium tuberculosis*
- (D) *Pseudomonas aeruginosa*
- * (E) *Staphylococcus aureus*

Vertebral osteomyelitis, or discitis, is a rare infection. The infection usually results from the hematogenous spread of a bacterial or yeast infection to vertebral bones and, subsequently, to the adjacent intervertebral disc space. However, it also can result from contiguous spread from an adjacent soft tissue infection or from direct inoculation from trauma or spinal surgery. Patients generally have progressively worsening back pain and possible lower extremity weakness. Physical examination findings include tenderness over the affected spine, generally with preserved neurologic function. Diagnosis is made with magnetic resonance imaging, which typically demonstrates significant enhancement and signal changes at the affected vertebrae and intervertebral space on T2-weighted imaging (Fig. 46-1). The infection may be initially treated with broad-spectrum antibiotics, but lack of response to conservative measures requires surgical debridement and possible reconstructive procedures.

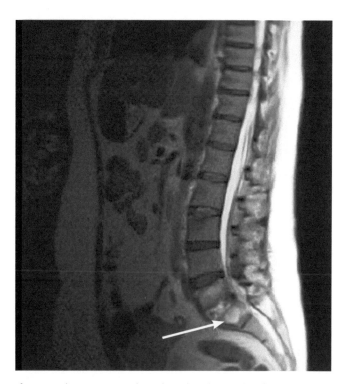

FIG. 46-1. Sagittal section of magnetic resonance imaging showing an L5–S1 discitis with an epidural abscess. (Muffly TM, Diwadkar GB, Paraiso MF. Lumbosacral osteomyelitis after robot-assisted total laparoscopic hysterectomy and sacral colpopexy. Int Urogynecol J 2010;21:1569–71.)

Although vertebral osteomyelitis after minimally invasive sacrocolpopexy is a rare complication, incidence rates are unknown and several case reports have been published. Sacrocolpopexy involves attachment of synthetic mesh to the vagina or cervix and the anterior longitudinal ligament as it runs over the sacral promontory. The infection is thought to result from direct communication and bacterial seeding from the vagina as well as deep placement of the sutures through the anterior longitudinal ligament and into the intervertebral disc. Recent studies have suggested that in the supine position, the most prominent structure in the presacral space is the L5–S1 intervertebral disc. In order to avoid possible placement of the stitch into the disc space, surgeons should place the suture at least 1–2 mm below the promontory drop before placing the suspension sutures (Fig. 46-2).

The most common pathogen isolated in cases of vertebral osteomyelitis associated with sacrocolpopexy is *S aureus*, although *C albicans* has been isolated in one case report. Group B *Streptococcus*, *M tuberculosis*, and *P aeruginosa* are less commonly isolated from associated abscesses. Therefore, the most likely microbial pathogen associated with the described patient's vertebral discitis is *S aureus*.

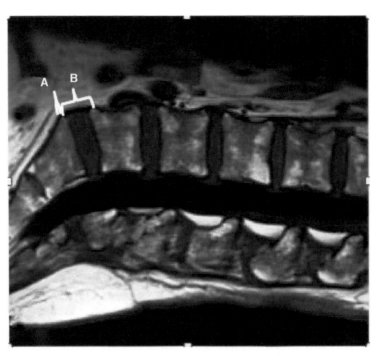

FIG. 46-2. Sagittal section of magnetic resonance imaging. **A.** Distance from bony promontory to base of L5–S1 intervertebral disc: 1 mm. **B.** Distance from bony promontory to base of L5: 13 mm. (Abernethy M, Vasquez E, Kenton K, Brubaker L, Mueller E. Where do we place the sacrocolpopexy stitch? A magnetic resonance imaging investigation. Female Pelvic Med Reconstr Surg 2013;19:31–3.)

Abernethy M, Vasquez E, Kenton K, Brubaker L, Mueller E. Where do we place the sacrocolpopexy stitch? A magnetic resonance imaging investigation. Female Pelvic Med Reconstr Surg 2013;19:31–3.

Beronius M, Bergman B, Andersson R. Vertebral osteomyelitis in Goteborg, Sweden: a retrospective study of patients during 1990–95. Scand J Infect Dis 2001;33:527–32.

Good MM, Abele TA, Balgobin S, Schaffer JI, Slocum P, McIntire D, et al. Preventing L5–S1 discitis associated with sacrocolpopexy. Obstet Gynecol 2013;121:285–90.

Kehrer M, Pedersen C, Jensen TG, Lassen AT. Increasing incidence of pyogenic spondylodiscitis: a 14-year population-based study. J Infect 2014;68:313–20.

Muffly TM, Diwadkar GB, Paraiso MF. Lumbosacral osteomyelitis after robot-assisted total laparoscopic hysterectomy and sacral colpopexy. Int Urogynecol J 2010;21:1569–71.

47

Nerve entrapment with uterosacral ligament suspension

A 74-year-old woman visits your office with a vaginal bulge she has felt for 6 months. She has experienced no urinary incontinence, retention, or bowel issues. She has no prior surgical history and has well-controlled diabetes mellitus. On examination, she has stage III uterine prolapse. She tried a pessary but did not like the maintenance required and instead has elected to undergo definitive surgical correction. After options counseling, she chooses to have a total vaginal hysterectomy with bilateral salpingo-oophorectomy and uterosacral ligament suspension. Postoperatively, she is experiencing pain and numbness in the left buttock that radiates down the back of her thigh to her popliteal fossa. No motor compromise is detected. The most likely cause of her pain and numbness is

(A) compression of the common peroneal nerve
* (B) entrapment of sacral nerve roots
(C) femoral neuropathy
(D) diabetic neuropathy

Surgical techniques to address apical support defects can be achieved through use of either a vaginal or abdominal approach. Such surgery can be performed through a traditional incision or a minimally invasive procedure. One vaginal approach is uterosacral ligament suspension, which is a native tissue repair.

A uterosacral ligament suspension usually follows vaginal hysterectomy or is performed after entry into the peritoneal cavity via a vaginal incision. While the ureter is retracted laterally and the rectum retracted medially, sutures are placed into the uterosacral ligament at the level of the ischial spine. Often, the location of the uterosacral ligament is confirmed by placing an Allis forceps on the vaginal cuff and applying traction to tent the uterosacral ligament to make it palpable and visible under the posterior peritoneum in the pelvis. If sutures are placed too lateral or too deeply, sacral nerve branches can be entrapped or even ligated, which will cause pain and numbness in the S2–S4 distribution.

If nerve entrapment is suspected based on the patient's symptoms, all permanent sutures should be removed immediately. If an absorbable suture was used, symptoms can be managed with narcotics and neuropathic pain medications, such as gabapentin, because time usually will resolve the symptoms. Some experts have suggested that elevating the uterosacral ligaments off the posterior pelvic wall with the use of Allis forceps will help prevent too deep of a bite with the placement of sutures.

The described patient has pain and numbness that radiates down the posterior leg, which is consistent with an S2–S4 distribution, or entrapment of sciatic nerves with the uterosacral stitch. The most likely cause of her pain and numbness is entrapment of sacral nerve roots.

Peroneal nerve injury usually is caused by improper positioning of the patient's legs in the stirrups in the operating room. Pressure on the lateral aspect of the fibula will compress the common peroneal nerve. Symptoms include foot drop, gait instability, and numbness over the lateral leg and dorsum of the feet.

Femoral neuropathy can be caused by positioning the patient in stirrups. Hyperflexion of the thigh can compress the nerve under the inguinal ligament. Femoral neuropathy can have sensory and motor components, specifically sensation loss in the anterior and medial thigh and weakness in the quadriceps and iliopsoas muscles, which causes difficulty flexing the hip and extending the knee. Diabetic neuropathy is primarily symmetrical and sensory and usually starts with the distal lower extremities in a typical "stocking-glove" pattern.

Flynn MK, Weidner AC, Amundsen CL. Sensory nerve injury after uterosacral ligament suspension. Am J Obstet Gynecol 2006;195: 1869–72.

Pelvic organ prolapse. ACOG Practice Bulletin No. 85. American College of Obstetricians and Gynecologists. Obstet Gynecol 2007;110: 717–29.

48

Electrosurgery

During a laparoscopic salpingo-oophorectomy, you use a bipolar electrosurgical energy source to secure the blood supply to the ovary within the infundibulopelvic ligament before transecting it. The correct term for the electrosurgical function you perform with the bipolar device is

     (A) cauterization
     (B) fulguration
     (C) vaporization
*   (D) coagulation

Although it is commonly used to describe electrosurgery, the term "cauterization" refers to the conduction of heat via direct current from a probe heated to a very high temperature. Examples include branding cattle, soldering iron, or grill lines on a steak. Electrosurgery is the use of alternating current produced by a generator and applied to the tissue with a handheld electrode in order to heat the tissue itself.

When electrosurgical current is applied in a very concentrated way at high voltage, the intense heat delivered to the tissue causes the fluid inside cells to vaporize and the cells to burst. A high voltage is required to push the current through the vapor. Vaporization is performed on cutting mode, which delivers continuous current without direct contact with the tissue. Vaporization avoids an eschar or coagulum, creating a clean wound with minimal necrotic tissue at the wound borders.

When electrosurgical current is applied to tissue over a relatively wide surface, the amount of heat generated is too low to vaporize the tissue. The tissue is increasingly heated at the surface, desiccating it and making it increasingly less conductive. This dry patch of dead tissue is called a coagulum. Fulguration is the process of creating a superficial coagulum by applying intermittent energy to a tissue surface using a monopolar electrode without direct tissue contact. In gynecology, this is commonly done with the rollerball attachment to the electrocautery device to stop cervical bleeding after a loop electrosurgical excision procedure.

Electrosurgical current also can be applied with direct tissue contact, causing a deeper coagulum. Bipolar electrosurgical devices contain the active electrode and the return electrode in their jaws. This serves to isolate the vascular pedicle clamped tissue between the jaws as the electrical circuit. As the tissue is heated, the collagen and elastin found in the blood vessel walls denature, forming a hemostatic coagulum. The bipolar generator measures the impedance of the tissue circuit as it delivers the current and shuts off when a certain impedance is reached, indicating that desiccation is complete.

Covidien Energy-based Professional Education. Principles in Electrosurgery. Available at: http://www.asit.org/assets/documents/ Prinicpals_in_electrosurgery.pdf. Accessed October 8, 2015.

Hainer BL. Fundamentals of electrosurgery. J Am Board Fam Pract 1991;4:419–26.

Massarweh NN, Cosgriff N, Slakey DP. Electrosurgery: history, principles, and current and future uses. J Am Coll Surg 2006;202:520–30.

49

Venous thromboembolism and perioperative thromboprophylaxis

A 57-year-old postmenopausal woman comes to your clinic for preoperative counseling. She has stage III uterovaginal prolapse and is scheduled to undergo a vaginal hysterectomy and uterosacral ligament suspension. Her weight is 90.7 kg (200 lb), and her body mass index (weight in kilograms divided by height in meters squared [kg/m^2]) is 37. She is otherwise healthy, has no history of venous thromboembolism, does not smoke, and takes combination hormone therapy. Based on the patient's presentation, her perioperative thromboprophylaxis should be

    (A) early ambulation
    (B) compression stockings
*   (C) intermittent pneumatic compression devices
    (D) enoxaparin twice daily

An important avoidable complication after reconstructive pelvic surgery is a thromboembolic event. Established risk factors for the development of a deep venous thromboembolism or pulmonary embolism include surgery and immobilization during the postoperative recovery period. Although such events are rare, with an incidence of 0.1–0.3%, they can be catastrophic. It is estimated that 50% of patients present with a fatal pulmonary embolism, and among individuals who survive, up to 90% will continue to have sequelae 2 years later. However, the morbidity and mortality is modifiable with the use of appropriate perioperative prophylaxis. Table 49-1 lists the American College of Obstetricians and Gynecologists guidelines for perioperative thromboembolic prophylaxis based on risk stratification. Following these guidelines, patients are stratified into one of four risk categories based on the length of surgery, age, and the presence of additional risk factors. Box 49-1 lists venous thromboembolism risk factors. The described patient would be considered to have a high risk of a thromboembolic event.

TABLE 49-1. Risk Classification for Venous Thromboembolism in Patients Undergoing Surgery Without Prophylaxis

Level of Risk	Definition	Successful Prevention Strategies
Low	Surgery lasting less than 30 minutes in patients younger than 40 years with no additional risk factors	No specific prophylaxis; early and "aggressive" mobilization
Moderate	Surgery lasting less than 30 minutes in patients with additional risk factors; surgery lasting less than 30 minutes in patients aged 40–60 years with no additional risk factors; major surgery in patients younger than 40 years with no additional risk factors	Low-dose unfractionated heparin (5,000 units every 12 hours), LMWH (2,500 units dalteparin or 40 mg enoxaparin daily), graduated compression stockings, or intermittent pneumatic compression devices
High	Surgery lasting less than 30 minutes in patients older than 60 years or with additional risk factors; major surgery in patients older than 40 years or with additional risk factors	Low-dose unfractionated heparin (5,000 units every 8 hours), LMWH (5,000 units dalteparin or 40 mg enoxaparin daily), graduated compression stockings, or intermittent pneumatic compression devices
Highest	Major surgery in patients older than 60 years plus prior venous thromboembolism, cancer, or molecular hypercoagulable state	Low-dose unfractionated heparin (5,000 units every 8 hours), LMWH (5,000 units dalteparin or 40 mg enoxaparin daily), graduated compression stockings, or intermittent pneumatic compression devices + low-dose unfractionated heparin or LMWH. Consider continuing prophylaxis for 2–4 weeks after discharge.

Abbreviation: LMWH, low-molecular-weight heparin.

Prevention of deep vein thrombosis and pulmonary embolism. ACOG Practice Bulletin No. 84. American College of Obstetricians and Gynecologists. Obstet Gynecol 2007;110:429–40.

BOX 49-1

Venous Thromboembolism Risk Factors

Surgery

Trauma (major or lower extremity)

Immobility, paresis

Malignancy

Cancer therapy (hormonal, chemotherapy, or radiotherapy)

Previous venous thromboembolism

Increasing age

Pregnancy and the postpartum period

Estrogen-containing oral contraception or hormone therapy

Selective estrogen receptor modulators

Acute medical illness

Heart or respiratory failure

Inflammatory bowel disease

Myeloproliferative disorders

Paroxysmal nocturnal hemoglobinuria

Nephrotic syndrome

Obesity

Smoking

Varicose veins

Central venous catheterization

Inherited or acquired thrombophilia

Prevention of deep vein thrombosis and pulmonary embolism. ACOG Practice Bulletin No. 84. American College of Obstetricians and Gynecologists. Obstet Gynecol 2007;110:429–40.

Following the guidelines, the appropriate perioperative order for the described patient would be for intermittent pneumatic compression devices. Although enoxaparin alone is an appropriate choice, the correct dosage is daily, not twice daily. This patient does not require dual prophylaxis, which is reserved for patients who are considered to be at highest risk.

Antibiotic prophylaxis for gynecologic procedures. ACOG Practice Bulletin No. 104. American College of Obstetricians and Gynecologists. Obstet Gynecol 2009;113:1180–9.

Gould MK, Garcia DA, Wren SM, Karanicolas PJ, Arcelus JI, Heit JA, et al. Prevention of VTE in nonorthopedic surgical patients: Antithrombotic Therapy and Prevention of Thrombosis, 9th ed: American College of Chest Physicians Evidence-Based Clinical Practice Guidelines. American College of Chest Physicians [published erratum appears in Chest 2012;141:1369]. Chest 2012;141:e227S–77S.

Guyatt GH, Akl EA, Crowther M, Gutterman DD, Schuunemann HJ. Executive summary: Antithrombotic Therapy and Prevention of Thrombosis, 9th ed: American College of Chest Physicians Evidence-Based Clinical Practice Guidelines. American College of Chest Physicians Antithrombotic Therapy and Prevention of Thrombosis Panel [published errata appear in Chest 2012;142:1698; Chest 2012;141:1129]. Chest 2012;141:7S–47S.

Mueller MG, Pilecki MA, Catanzarite T, Jain U, Kim JY, Kenton K. Venous thromboembolism in reconstructive pelvic surgery. Am J Obstet Gynecol 2014;211:552.e1–6.

Prevention of deep vein thrombosis and pulmonary embolism. ACOG Practice Bulletin No. 84. American College of Obstetricians and Gynecologists. Obstet Gynecol 2007;110:429–40.

Solomon ER, Frick AC, Paraiso MF, Barber MD. Risk of deep venous thrombosis and pulmonary embolism in urogynecologic surgical patients. Am J Obstet Gynecol 2010;203:510.e1–4.

50

Midurethral slings

A 42-year-old multiparous woman has urinary leakage with coughing, sneezing, and exercise. She tried an incontinence pessary in the past without improvement in her symptoms. Her anterior vaginal wall comes to the hymen and she has urethral hypermobility. Her cough stress test result is positive. After discussing the nonsurgical and surgical options, she is eager for definitive management and wants the treatment with highest success rate and shortest recovery time. The most appropriate treatment for this patient is

   (A) autologous fascial sling
   (B) onabotulinumtoxinA
 * (C) midurethral sling
   (D) urethral bulking agent
   (E) physical therapy

Midurethral slings were introduced in the 1990s and are the primary surgical treatment for stress urinary incontinence in women. Reports estimate a 27% increase in the surgical management of stress urinary incontinence from 2000 to 2009, most of which is secondary to an increase in the number of sling procedures. A meta-analysis of 62 randomized trials concluded that midurethral slings are as effective as Burch colposuspension and fascial slings but are associated with shorter operative times, quicker recovery, and fewer postoperative complications. Short-term cure rates for midurethral slings were found to be comparable to fascial sling (73% versus 71%, respectively), open Burch colposuspension (79% versus 82%, respectively), and laparoscopic colposuspension (82% versus 74%, respectively), although none of these differences was statistically significant. Rates of new-onset urgency and urgency incontinence are lower after midurethral sling compared with fascial slings.

Several large multicenter trials compared retropubic with transobturator midurethral slings. The Trial of Mid-Urethral Slings randomized women with stress urinary incontinence to retropubic or transobturator midurethral slings. Using a composite primary outcome (negative cough stress test, negative pad test, no retreatment, no self-reported symptoms, and no leakage episodes on voiding diary), the procedures were equivalent at 1 year (81% for retropubic slings and 78% for transobturator slings). However, at 2 years and 5 years after surgery, neither objective nor subjective success rates met the predefined criteria for equivalence. Voiding dysfunction was more common with retropubic slings (2.7% versus 0.0%), but neurologic symptoms were more common with transobturator slings (9.4% versus 4.0%). The most common adverse effect was urinary tract infection (26%). Mesh complications (3.4%) were uncommon (16 exposures and 2 erosions). The described patient is young with

uncomplicated primary stress incontinence and desires a permanent procedure with a quick recovery. Thus, a midurethral sling is the best management for her.

For patients who decline synthetic mesh slings or who are not candidates for such mesh slings, autologous fascial slings are an effective treatment option. Given the higher rates of voiding dysfunction, urinary tract infections, and longer recovery times associated with fascial slings, a fascial sling is not the first-line choice for the described patient. A fascial sling may be considered for the treatment of stress incontinence in a woman with a nonmobile, fixed urethra secondary to its more obstructive nature. In addition, a fascial sling can be placed under more tension (more obstructive) than a synthetic sling secondary to the risks of urethral erosion with a synthetic sling. Additionally, a woman who had complications from prior mesh placed in the anterior vagina (for sling or prolapse) may be a candidate for the autologous fascial sling. Several case series report good outcomes with removal of prior mesh and placement of an autologous fascial sling.

OnabotulinumtoxinA is effective for the treatment of urgency urinary incontinence in women who do not respond to more conservative treatments, cannot tolerate adverse effects associated with antimuscarinic agents, or who do not want to take a daily medication. In a recent double-blind, randomized comparative effectiveness trial, women with urgency urinary incontinence were assigned to intravesical onabotulinumtoxinA plus placebo pills or antimuscarinic medications plus placebo injection in the bladder. Forty-one percent of participants were naïve to antimuscarinic therapy and none had previously tried more than two anticholinergic agents. The treatments resulted in similar reductions in daily incontinence episodes at 6 months (3.3 and 3.4, respectively); however, 27% of women in the onabotulinumtoxinA arm, compared with only 13% in the antimuscarinic arm, were completely dry. Because the described patient has stress incontinence and not urgency incontinence, onabotulinumtoxinA would not be the best choice for her.

Urethral bulking agents are not recommended as a primary treatment for stress urinary incontinence but remain an option for women with persistent stress urinary incontinence or women with comorbidities who cannot tolerate anesthesia or surgery. A Cochrane review found that urethral bulking agents are less effective than slings, with 1.7–4.7-fold increased likelihood of cure with surgical treatment.

Although pelvic floor muscle exercises (ie, Kegel exercises) are an effective treatment for stress incontinence, the efficacy of such treatment decreases over time. A recent randomized comparative effectiveness trial compared midurethral sling with pelvic floor physical therapy for treatment of primary stress urinary incontinence and allowed for crossover between the study groups. The investigators observed higher subjective and objective cure rates among the women who received the midurethral sling. Subjective improvement was reported by 91% of the women after midurethral sling and 64% after physical therapy (absolute difference, 26.4%; 95% confidence interval, 18.1–34.5). It was found that 49% of women in the physical therapy group crossed over and underwent midurethral sling surgery compared with only 11% in the midurethral sling group transferring to physical therapy. Therefore, for this patient who desires definitive management with the highest efficacy, physical therapy would not be the best choice.

Albo ME, Litman HJ, Richter HE, Lemack GE, Sirls LT, Chai TC, et al. Treatment success of retropubic and transobturator mid urethral slings at 24 months. J Urol 2012;188:2281–7.

Anger JT, Weinberg AE, Albo ME, Smith AL, Kim JH, Rodriguez LV, et al. Trends in surgical management of stress urinary incontinence among female Medicare beneficiaries. Urology 2009;74:283–7.

Barber MD, Kleeman S, Karram MM, Paraiso MF, Walters MD, Vasavada S, et al. Transobturator tape compared with tension-free vaginal tape for the treatment of stress urinary incontinence: a randomized controlled trial. Obstet Gynecol 2008;111:611–21.

Blaivas JG, Purohit RS, Weinberger JM, Tsui JF, Chouhan J, Sidhu R, et al. Salvage surgery after failed treatment of synthetic mesh sling complications. J Urol 2013;190:1281–6.

Dumoulin C, Hay-Smith EJC, Mac Habée-Séguin G. Pelvic floor muscle training versus no treatment, or inactive control treatments, for urinary incontinence in women. Cochrane Database of Systematic Reviews 2014, Issue 5. Art. No.: CD005654. DOI: 10.1002/14651858. CD005654.pub3.

Ford AA, Rogerson L, Cody JD, Ogah J. Mid-urethral sling operations for stress urinary incontinence in women. Cochrane Database of Systematic Reviews 2015, Issue 7. Art. No.: CD006375. DOI: 10.1002/14651858.CD006375.pub3.

Jonsson Funk M, Levin PJ, Wu JM. Trends in the surgical management of stress urinary incontinence. Obstet Gynecol 2012;119:845–51.

Kirchin V, Page T, Keegan PE, Atiemo K, Cody JD, McClinton S. Urethral injection therapy for urinary incontinence in women. Cochrane Database of Systematic Reviews 2012, Issue 2. Art. No.: CD003881. DOI: 10.1002/14651858.CD003881.pub3.

Labrie J, Berghmans BL, Fischer K, Milani AL, van der Wijk I, Smalbraak DJ, et al. Surgery versus physiotherapy for stress urinary incontinence. N Engl J Med 2013;369:1124–33.

Richter HE, Albo ME, Zyczynski HM, Kenton K, Norton PA, Sirls LT, et al. Retropubic versus transobturator midurethral slings for stress incontinence. Urinary Incontinence Treatment Network. N Engl J Med 2010;362:2066–76.

Richter HE, Burgio KL, Brubaker L, Nygaard IE, Ye W, Weidner A, et al. Continence pessary compared with behavioral therapy or combined therapy for stress incontinence: a randomized controlled trial. Pelvic Floor Disorders Network. Obstet Gynecol 2010;115:609–17.

Shah K, Nikolavsky D, Gilsdorf D, Flynn BJ. Surgical management of lower urinary mesh perforation after mid-urethral polypropylene mesh sling: mesh excision, urinary tract reconstruction and concomitant pubovaginal sling with autologous rectus fascia. Int Urogynecol J 2013;24:2111–7.

Visco AG, Brubaker L, Richter HE, Nygaard I, Paraiso MF, Menefee SA, et al. Anticholinergic versus botulinum toxin A comparison trial for the treatment of bothersome urge urinary incontinence: ABC trial. Contemp Clin Trials 2012;33:184–96.

Appendix A
Normal Values for Laboratory Tests*

Analyte	Conventional Units
Alanine aminotransferase, serum	8–35 units/L
Alkaline phosphatase, serum	15–120 units/L
Menopause	
Amniotic fluid index	3–30 mL
Amylase	20–300 units/L
Greater than 60 years old	21–160 units/L
Aspartate aminotransferase, serum	15–30 units/L
Bicarbonate	
Arterial blood	21–27 mEq/L
Venous plasma	23–29 mEq/L
Bilirubin	
Total	0.3–1 mg/dL
Conjugated (direct)	0.1–0.4 mg/dL
Newborn, total	1–10 mg/dL
Blood gases (arterial) and pulmonary function	
Base deficit	Less than 3 mEq/L
Base excess, arterial blood, calculated	–2 mEq/L to +3 mEq/L
Forced expiratory volume (FEV_1)	3.5–5 L
	Greater than 80% of predicted value
Forced vital capacity	3.5–5 L
Oxygen saturation (Sao_2)	95% or higher
Pao_2	80 mm Hg or more
Pco_2	35–45 mm Hg
Po_2	80–95 mm Hg
Peak expiratory flow rate	Approximately 450 L/min
pH	7.35–7.45
Pvo_2	30–40 mm Hg
Blood urea nitrogen	
Adult	7–18 mg/dL
Greater than 60 years old	8–20 mg/dL
CA 125	Less than 34 units/mL
Calcium	
Ionized	4.6–5.3 mg/dL
Serum	8.6–10 mg/dL
Chloride	98–106 mEq/L
Cholesterol	
Total	
Desirable	140–199 mg/dL
Borderline high	200–239 mg/dL
High	240 mg/dL or more
High-density lipoprotein	40–85 mg/dL
Low-density lipoprotein	
Desirable	Less than 130 mg/dL
Borderline high	140–159 mg/dL
High	Greater than 160 mg/dL
Total cholesterol-to-high-density lipoprotein ratio	
Desirable	Less than 3
Borderline high	3–5
High	Greater than 5
Triglycerides	
20 years and older	Less than 150 mg/dL
Younger than 20 years old	35–135 mg/dL

*Values listed are specific for adults or women, if relevant, unless otherwise differentiated.

(continued)

Normal Values for Laboratory Tests* (*continued*)

Analyte	Conventional Units
Cortisol, plasma	
8 AM	5–23 micrograms/dL
4 PM	3–15 micrograms/dL
10 PM	Less than 50% of 8 AM value
Creatinine, serum	0.6–1.2 mg/dL
Dehydroepiandrosterone sulfate	60–340 micrograms/dL
Erythrocyte	
Count	3,800,000–5,100,000/mm^3
Distribution width	10 plus or minus 1.5%
Sedimentation rate	
Wintrobe method	0–15 mm/hour
Westergren method	0–20 mm/hour
Estradiol-17β	
Follicular phase	30–100 pg/mL
Ovulatory phase	200–400 pg/mL
Luteal phase	50–140 pg/mL
Child	0.8–56 pg/mL
Ferritin, serum	18–160 micrograms/L
Fibrinogen	150–400 mg/dL
Follicle-stimulating hormone	
Premenopause	2.8–17.2 mIU/mL
Midcycle peak	15–35 mIU/mL
Postmenopause	24–170 mIU/mL
Child	0.1–7 mIU/mL
Glucose	
Fasting	70–105 mg/dL
2-hour postprandial	Less than 120 mg/dL
Random blood	65–110 mg/dL
Hematocrit	36–48%
Hemoglobin	12–16 g/dL
Fetal	Less than 1% of total
Hemoglobin A$_{1c}$ (nondiabetic)	5.5–8.5%
Human chorionic gonadotropin	0–5 mIU/mL
Pregnant	Greater than 5 mIU/mL
17α-Hydroxyprogesterone	
Adult	50–300 ng/dL
Child	32–63 ng/dL
25-Hydroxyvitamin D	10–55 ng/mL
International Normalized Ratio	Greater than 1
Prothrombin time	10–13 seconds
Iron, serum	65–165 micrograms/dL
Binding capacity total	240–450 micrograms/dL
Lactate dehydrogenase, serum	313–618 units/L
Leukocytes	
Total	5,000–10,000/cubic micrometers
Differential counts	
Basophils	0–1%
Eosinophils	1–3%
Lymphocytes	25–33%
Monocytes	3–7%
Myelocytes	0%
Band neutrophils	3–5%
Segmented neutrophils	54–62%

*Values listed are specific for adults or women, if relevant, unless otherwise differentiated.

(*continued*)

Normal Values for Laboratory Tests* (*continued*)

Analyte	Conventional Units
Lipase	
60 years or younger	10–140 units/L
Older than 60 years	18–180 units/L
Luteinizing hormone	
Follicular phase	3.6–29.4 mIU/mL
Midcycle peak	58–204 mIU/mL
Postmenopause	35–129 mIU/mL
Child	0.5–10.3 mIU/mL
Magnesium	
Adult	1.6–2.6 mg/dL
Child	1.7–2.1 mg/dL
Newborn	1.5–2.2 mg/dL
Mean corpuscular	
mCH Hemoglobin	27–33 pg
mCHC Hemoglobin concentration	33–37 g/dL
mCV Volume	80–100 cubic micrometers
Partial thromboplastin time, activated	21–35 seconds
Phosphate, inorganic phosphorus	2.5–4.5 mg/dL
Platelet count	140,000–400,000/mm^3
Potassium	3.5–5.3 mEq/L
Progesterone	
Follicular phase	Less than 3 ng/mL
Luteal phase	2.5–28 ng/mL
On oral contraceptives	0.1–0.3 ng/mL
Secretory phase	5–30 ng/mL
Older than 60 years	0–0.2 ng/mL
1st trimester	9–47 ng/mL
2nd trimester	16.8–146 ng/mL
3rd trimester	55–255 ng/mL
Prolactin	0–17 ng/mL
Pregnant	34–386 ng/mL by 3rd trimester
Prothrombin time	10–13 seconds
Reticulocyte count	Absolute: 25,000–85,000 cubic micrometers
	0.5–2.5% of erythrocytes
Semen analysis, spermatozoa	
Antisperm antibody	% of sperm binding by immunobead technique; greater than 20% = decreased fertility
Count	Greater than or equal to 20 million/mL
Motility	Greater than or equal to 50%
Morphology	Greater than or equal to 15% normal forms
Sodium	135–145 mEq/L
Testosterone, female	
Total	6–86 ng/dL
Pregnant	3–4 × normal
Postmenopause	One half of normal
Free	
20–29 years old	0.9–3.2 pg/mL
30–39 years old	0.8–3 pg/mL
40–49 years old	0.6–2.5 pg/mL
50–59 years old	0.3–2.7 pg/mL
Older than 60 years	0.2–2.2 pg/mL
Thyroid-stimulating hormone	0.2–3 microunits/mL
Thyroxine	
Serum free	0.9–2.3 ng/dL
Total	1.5–4.5 micrograms/dL

*Values listed are specific for adults or women, if relevant, unless otherwise differentiated.

(*continued*)

Normal Values for Laboratory Tests* (*continued*)

Analyte	Conventional Units
Triiodothyronine uptake	25–35%
Urea nitrogen, blood	
Adult	7–18 mg/dL
Older than 60 years	8–20 mg/dL
Uric acid, serum	2.6–6 mg/dL
Urinalysis	
Epithelial cells	0–3/HPF
Erythrocytes	0–3/HPF
Leukocytes	0–4/HPF
Protein (albumin)	
Qualitative	None detected
Quantitative	10–100 mg/24 hours
Pregnancy	Less than 300 mg/24 hours
Urine specific gravity	
Normal hydration and volume	1.005–1.03
Concentrated	1.025–1.03
Diluted	1.001–1.01

*Values listed are specific for adults or women, if relevant, unless otherwise differentiated.

Index

NOTE: Numbers refer to questions, not pages.

NOTE: Numbers refer to questions, not pages.

NOTE: Numbers refer to questions, not pages.

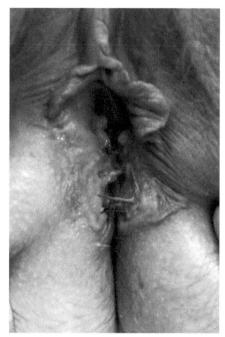

FIG. 4-1. Complete breakdown of wound. (Courtesy of Catherine Matthews, MD.)

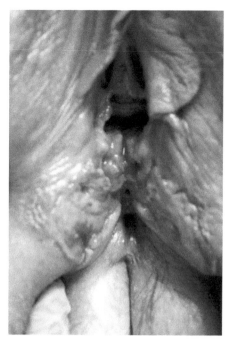

FIG. 4-2. Wound debrided. (Courtesy of Catherine Matthews, MD.)

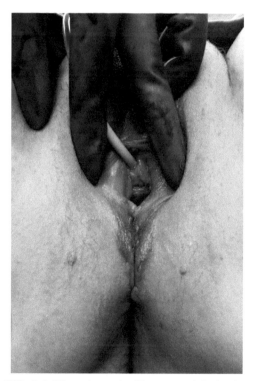

FIG. 4-3. Wound repair. (Courtesy of Catherine Matthews, MD.)

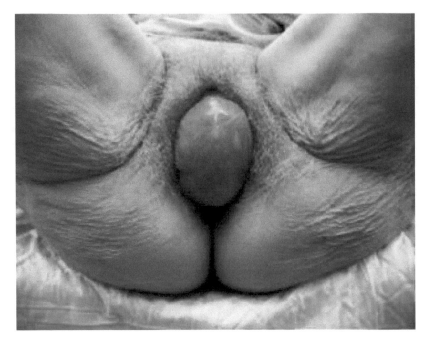

FIG. 7-1. Stage III pelvic organ prolapse. (Courtesy of Kimberly Kenton, MD.)

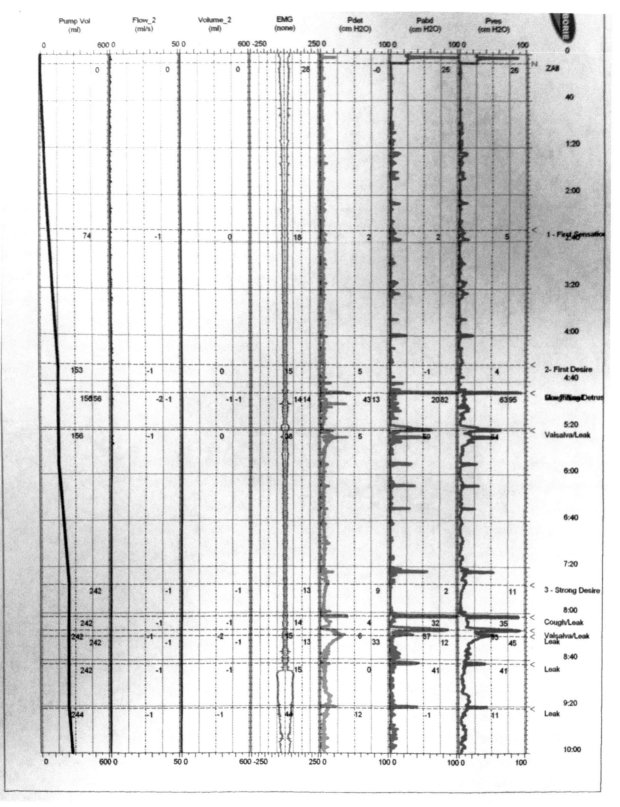

FIG. 9-1.

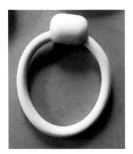

FIG. 11-1. Incontinence ring. The pessary is placed in the vagina so that the knob sits under the urethra, increasing urethral resistance. (Courtesy of Kimberly Kenton, MD.)

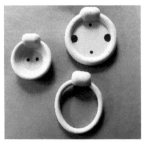

FIG. 11-2. Selection of incontinence pessaries. (Courtesy of Kimberly Kenton, MD.)

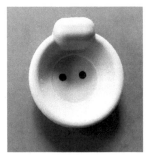

FIG. 11-3. Incontinence dish with support. (Courtesy of Kimberly Kenton, MD.)

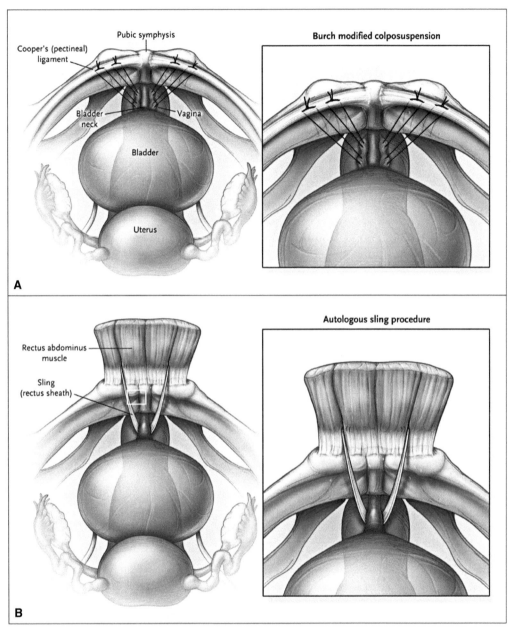

FIG. 12-1. Burch modified colposuspension and autologous sling procedure. In the Burch procedure **(A)**, permanent sutures are placed in the anterior vaginal wall at the level of the bladder neck and proximal urethra and are then sutured to the iliopectineal ligament. In the autologous sling procedure **(B)**, a strip of rectus fascia is harvested, and permanent sutures are placed at its two ends. The sling is placed beneath the proximal urethra through a vaginal incision. The two ends of the sling are passed behind the pubic bone to the anterior abdominal wall, where they are secured, either to each other or to the rectus fascia. (Albo ME, Richter HE, Brubaker L, Norton P, Kraus SR, Zimmern PE, et al. Burch colposuspension versus fascial sling to reduce urinary stress incontinence. Urinary Incontinence Treatment Network. N Engl J Med 2007;356:2143–55. Copyright 2007 by the Massachusetts Medical Society.)

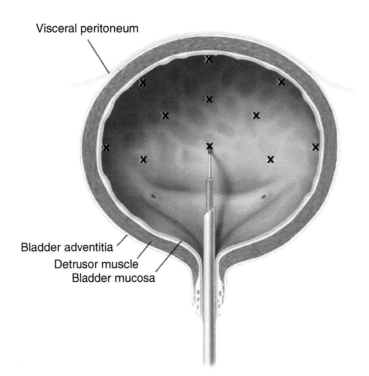

Visceral peritoneum

Bladder adventitia
Detrusor muscle
Bladder mucosa

FIG. 14-1. Botulinum-A neurotoxin injection into the detrusor muscle. (Reproduced with permission from Mahajan ST. Use of botulinum toxin for treatment of non-neurogenic lower urinary tract conditions. In: UpToDate, Post TW, Editor, UpToDate, Waltham, MA. Accessed on October 2, 2015. Copyright 2015 UpToDate, Inc. For more information visit http://www.uptodate.com.)

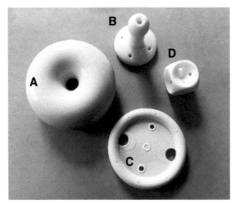

FIG. 20-1. Prolapse pessaries: **A.** Donut, **B.** Gellhorn, **C.** Ring with support, and **D.** Cube. (Courtesy of Kimberly Kenton, MD.)

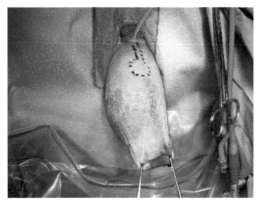

FIG. 20-2. Stage IV uterovaginal prolapse. The position of the urethrovesical junction is outlined on the vaginal epithelium, mimicking the location of the Foley balloon. (Courtesy of Kimberly Kenton, MD.)

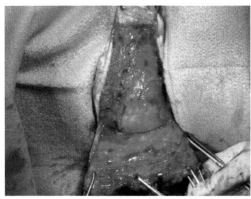

FIG. 20-3. The next step in colpocleisis is dissection of the posterior vaginal epithelium from the underlying endopelvic tissues. (Courtesy of Kimberly Kenton, MD.)

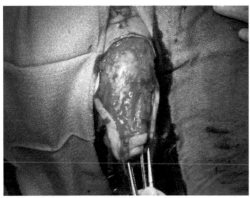

FIG. 20-4. The anterior vaginal epithelium is similarly removed. (Courtesy of Kimberly Kenton, MD.)

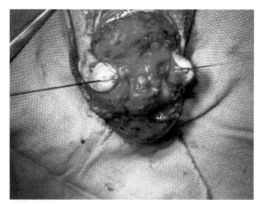

FIG. 20-5.

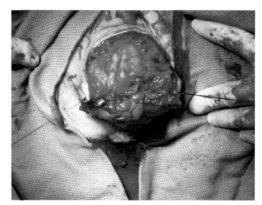

FIG. 20-6.

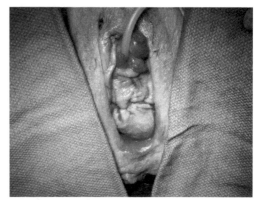

FIG. 20-7.

FIG. 20-5, FIG. 20-6, and FIG. 20-7. Serial imbricating sutures are placed across the anterior and posterior endopelvic connective tissues to reduce the uterus and prolapse. (Courtesy of Kimberly Kenton, MD.)

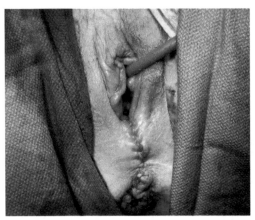

FIG. 20-8. View of colpocleisis after completion of perineorrhaphy, which significantly reduces the size of the genital hiatus. (Courtesy of Kimberly Kenton, MD.)

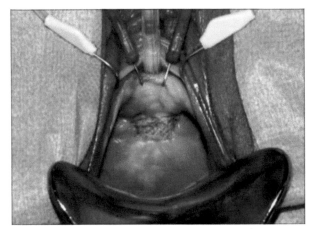

FIG. 22-1.

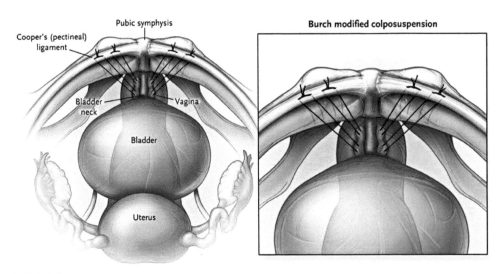

FIG. 23-1.

CATEGORY

	General Description	A (Asymptomatic)	B (Symptomatic)	C (Infection) D (Abscess)
1	**Vaginal:** no epithelial separation Include prominence (e.g. due to wrinkling or folding), penetration (without separation) or contraction (shrinkage) Grades of mesh contraction (*a-e*) from Table 4 is incorporated	1A: Abnormal prosthesis or graft finding on clinical examination	1B: Symptomatic e.g. unusual discomfort / pain; dyspareunia (either partner); bleeding	1C: Infection (suspected or actual)
2	**Vaginal:** smaller ≤ 1cm exposure	2A: Asymptomatic	2B: Symptomatic	2C: Infection D = Abscess
3	**Vaginal:** larger >1cm exposure, including extrusion	3A: Asymptomatic 1-3Aa if mesh contraction	3B: Symptomatic 1-3B (*b-e*) if mesh contraction	3C: Infection D = Abscess 1-3C (*b-e*) if mesh contraction
4	**Urinary Tract** compromise or perforation Include prosthesis (graft) perforation, fistula and calculus	4A: Small intraoperative defect e.g. bladder perforation	4B: Other lower urinary tract complication or urinary retention	4C: Ureteric or upper urinary tract complication
5	**Rectum or Bowel** compromise or perforation Include prosthesis (graft) perforation and fistula	5A: Small intraoperative defect (rectal or bowel)	5B: Rectal injury or compromise	5C: Small or Large bowel injury or compromise D = Abscess
6	**Skin** compromise Include discharge pain lump or sinus tract formation	6A: Asymptomatic, abnormal finding on clinical examination	6B: Symptomatic e.g. discharge, pain or lump	6C: Infection e.g. sinus tract formation D = Abscess
7	**Patient** compromise Include hematoma or systemic compromise	7A: Bleeding complication including haematoma	7B: Major degree of resuscitation or intensive care*	7C: Mortality * *(additional complication - no site applicable - S0)

TIME (clinically diagnosed)

T1: Intraoperative to 48 hours	T2: 48 hours to 6 months	T3: over 6 months

SITE

S1: Vaginal: area of suture line	S2: Vaginal: away from from area of suture line	S3: Trocar passage Exception: Intra-abdominal (S5)	S4: other skin site	S5: Intra-abdominal

N.B.   1. Multiple complications may occur in the same patient. There may be early and late complications in the same patient. i.e. All complications to be listed. Tables of complications may often be procedure specific.
2. The highest final category for any single complication should be used if there is a change within time. (patient 888)
3. Urinary tract infections and functional issues (apart from 4B) have not been included.

IUGA♀ ICS

☐☐☐ - T ☐ - S ☐

FIG. 27-1. A classification of complications related directly to the insertion of prostheses (meshes, implants, tapes) or grafts in urogynecologic surgery. (Haylen BT, Freeman RM, Swift SE, Cosson M, Davila GW, Deprest J, et al. An International Urogynecological Association [IUGA]/International Continence Society [ICS] joint terminology and classification of the complications related directly to the insertion of prostheses [meshes, implants, tapes] and grafts in female pelvic floor surgery. International Urogynecological Association, International Continence Society, and Joint IUGA/ICS Working Group on Complications Terminology. Neurourol Urodyn 2011;30:2–12.)

SACROCOLPOPEXY

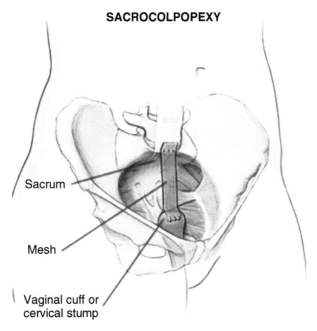

Sacrum

Mesh

Vaginal cuff or cervical stump

FIG. 28-1.

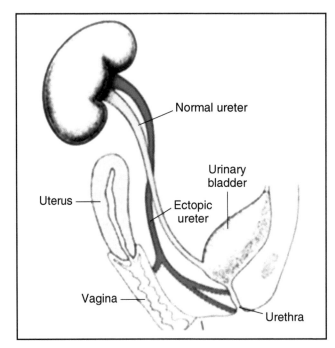

FIG. 32-1. Common sites for ectopic ureter in females. (Sadler TW. Urogenital system. In: Langman's medical embryology. 13th ed. Philadelphia (PA): Wolters Kluwer Health; 2015. p. 250–77.)

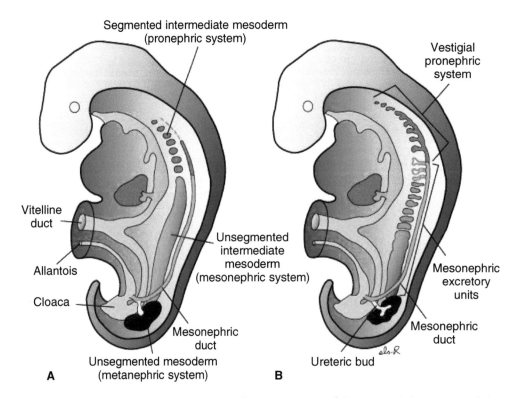

FIG. 32-2. A. Relationship of the intermediate mesoderm of the pronephric, mesonephric, and metanephric systems. In the lower thoracic, lumbar, and sacral regions, the intermediate mesoderm forms a solid, unsegmented mass of tissue, the nephrogenic cord. Note the longitudinal collecting duct, formed initially by the pronephros but later by the mesonephros (mesonephric duct). **B.** Excretory tubules of the pronephric and mesonephric systems in a 5-week embryo. (Sadler TW. Urogenital system. In: Langman's medical embryology. 13th ed. Philadelphia (PA): Wolters Kluwer Health; 2015. p. 250–77.)

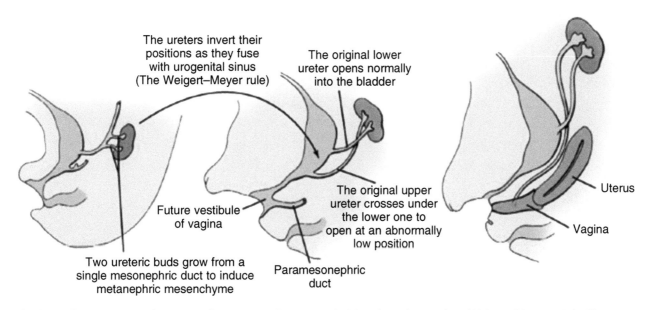

The ureters invert their positions as they fuse with urogenital sinus (The Weigert–Meyer rule)

The original lower ureter opens normally into the bladder

Future vestibule of vagina

The original upper ureter crosses under the lower one to open at an abnormally low position

Two ureteric buds grow from a single mesonephric duct to induce metanephric mesenchyme

Paramesonephric duct

Uterus

Vagina

FIG. 32-3. Development of an ectopic upper pole ureter draining into the vagina (Weigert–Meyer rule). (Sadler TW. Urogenital system. In: Langman's medical embryology. 13th ed. Philadelphia (PA): Wolters Kluwer Health; 2015. p. 250–77.)

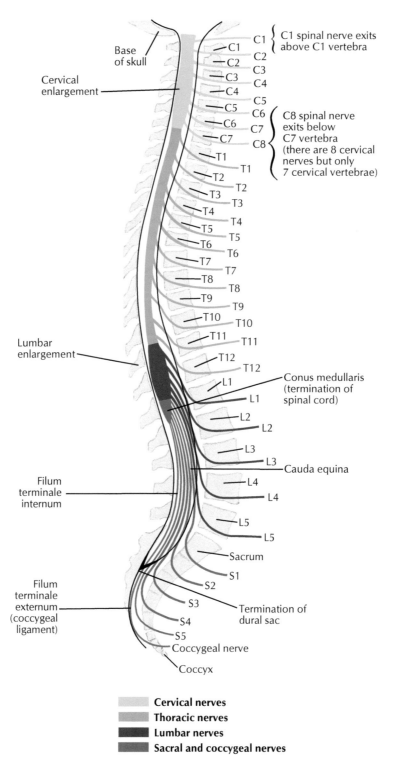

FIG. 34-1. Spinal cord and column levels showing nerve roots. (Netter FH. Atlas of human anatomy: with student consult access. 5th ed. New York (NY): W. B. Saunders, 2010.)

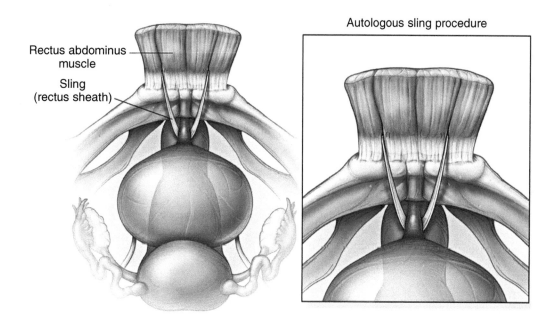

Rectus abdominus muscle

Sling (rectus sheath)

Autologous sling procedure

FIG. 35-1. Fascial sling. (Richter HE, Albo ME, Zyczynski HM, Kenton K, Norton PA, Sirls LT, et al. Retropubic versus transobturator I slings for stress incontinence. Urinary Incontinence Treatment Network. N Engl J Med 2010;362:2066–76. Copyright 2010 by the Massachusetts Medical Society.)

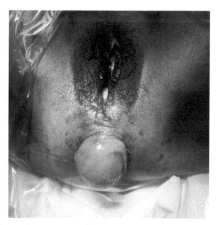

FIG. 41-1. Rectal prolapse. (Courtesy of Kimberly Kenton, MD.)

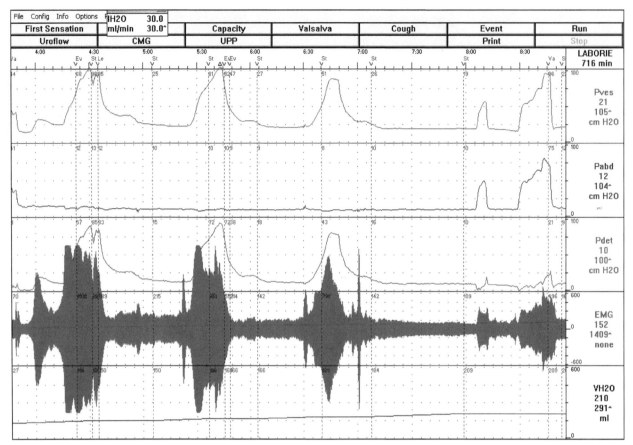

FIG. 43-1.

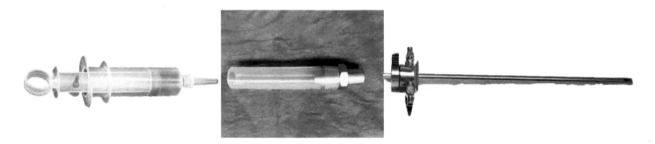

FIG. 44-1. Toomey adapter. (Courtesy of Kimberly Kenton, MD.)

Acknowledgments

FIG. 9-1. Courtesy of William Stuart Reynolds, MD, Department of Urologic Surgery, Vanderbilt University Medical Center, Nashville, TN.

Fig. 22-1 was originally published in Nazemi TM, Kobashi KC. Complications of grafts used in female pelvic floor reconstruction: mesh erosion and extrusion. Indian J Urol 2007;23:153–60.

Fig. 43-1 is provided courtesy of David Ginsberg, MD, Department of Urology, University of Southern California Institute of Urology, Los Angeles, CA.